Handbook of Chronic Total Occlusions

T0174378

Handbook of Chronic Total Occlusions

Edited by

George D Dangas MD PhD
Associate Professor of Medicine
Director of Postgraduate Training
Program Director, Interventional Cardiology
Columbia University Medical Center
Cardiovascular Research Foundation
New York, NY
USA

Roxana Mehran MD
Associate Professor of Medicine
Director, Outcomes Research
Data Coordination and Analysis Center
    for Interventional Vascular Therapy
Columbia University Medical Center
Cardiovascular Research Foundation
New York, NY
USA

Jeffrey W Moses MD
Professor of Medicine
Director, Center for Interventional Vascular Therapy
Columbia University Medical Center
Cardiovascular Research Foundation
New York, NY
USA

Foreword by

Martin B Leon

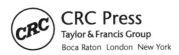

CRC Press
Taylor & Francis Group
Boca Raton London New York

CRC Press is an imprint of the
Taylor & Francis Group, an **informa** business

First published 2007 by Informa UK Ltd

Published 2019 by CRC Press
Taylor & Francis Group
6000 Broken Sound Parkway NW, Suite 300
Boca Raton, FL 33487-2742

© 2007 by Taylor & Francis Group, LLC
CRC Press is an imprint of Taylor & Francis Group, an Informa business

First issued in paperback 2019

No claim to original U.S. Government works

ISBN-13: 978-0-367-45295-7 (pbk)
ISBN-13: 978-1-84184-624-8 (hbk)

**Visit the Taylor & Francis Web site at
http://www.taylorandfrancis.com**

**and the CRC Press Web site at
http://www.crcpress.com**

A CIP record for this book is available from the British Library.
Library of Congress Cataloging-in-Publication Data

Contents

Contributors

Amr E Abbas MD
William Beaumont Hospital
Royal Oak, MI
USA

M Ishti Ali MD
St Joseph's Hospital and Medical
Center
Phoenix Heart Center
Phoenix, AZ
USA

Steven R Bailey MD
University of Texas Health Science
Center at San Antonio
San Antonio, TX
USA

Stephen Balter PhD
New York-Presbyterian Hospital
Columbia University Medical Center
New York, NY
USA

Gregory A Braden MD
Cardiology Specialists of North
Carolina
Winston-Salem, North Carolina
USA

Antonio Colombo MD
Columbus Hospital/San Raffaele
Hospital
Milan
Italy

George D Dangas MD PhD
Columbia University Medical Center
Cardiovascular Research Foundation
New York, NY
USA

Neil K Goyal MD MPH
Columbia University Medical Center
New York, NY
USA

William Gray MD
Columbia University Medical Center
Cardiovascular Research Foundation
New York, NY
USA

Richard Heuser MD
St Joseph's Hospital and Medical
Center
Phoenix Heart Center
Phoenix, Arizona
USA

Angela Hoye MB ChB PhD MRCP
Department of Cardiology
Castle Hill Hospital
Kingston-upon-Hull
UK

David E Kandzari MD
Duke Clinical Research Institute
Chapel Hill, NC
USA

Osamu Katoh MD
Toyohashi Heart Center
Toyohashi,
Aichi
Japan

Masashi Kimura MD PhD
Cardiovascular Research
Foundation
New York, NY
USA

Ajay J Kirtane MD
Columbia University Medical Center
Cardiovascular Research Foundation
New York, NY
USA

Roxana Mehran MD
Columbia University Medical Center
Cardiovascular Research Foundation
New York, NY
USA

Jeffrey W Moses MD
Columbia University Medical Center
Cardiovascular Research Foundation
New York, NY
USA

Eugenia Nikolsky MD PhD
University of Haifa
Haifa
Israel

Masahiko Ochiai MD PhD
Professor, Division of Cardiology
and Cardiovascular Surgery
Showa University Northern
Yokohama Hospital
Yokohama
Kanagawa
Japan

William W O'Neill MD
University of Miami
Florida
USA

Charles Perry MD MBA
Columbia University Medical Center
New York, NY
USA

Matthew J Price MD
Division of Cardiology
Scripps Clinic
La Jolla, California
USA

Mark Reisman MD
Swedish Heart Institute
Seattle, Washington
USA

Matthew Selmon MD
The Cleveland Clinic Foundation
Cleveland, Ohio
USA

Goran Stankovic MD
Institute for Cardiovascular Disease
Clinical Center of Serbia
Belgrade
Serbia

Jean-François Surmely MD
Swiss Cardiovascular Center
Bem University
Bem
Switzerland

Paul S Teirstein MD
Division of Cardiology
Scripps Clinic
La Jolla, California
USA

Etsuo Tsuchikane MD PhD
Toyohashi Heart Center
Toyohashi
Aichi
Japan

Patrick L Whitlow MD
The Cleveland Clinic Foundation
Cleveland, Ohio
USA

Garrett B Wong MD
Division of Cardiology
Scripps Clinic
La Jolla, California
USA

Foreword

The challenge of revascularizing chronic total coronary occlusions (CTO) has plagued the practicing interventionalist since the inception of coronary angioplasty, almost three decades ago. The presence of a CTO remains the single most frequent reason given for patient referral for coronary bypass surgery, as predictable revascularization success utilizing transcatheter techniques has been disappointing and treatment site recurrence (restenosis and re-occlusion) has been excessive. Nevertheless, there are growing data which indicate that successful treatment of CTOs results in improved symptoms, prolonged life, increased left ventricular function, and enhanced quality of life.

Importantly, significant changes have occurred over the past several years which have stimulated an energized re-examination of CTO therapy. First, the advent and use of drug-eluting stents has markedly reduced angiographic and clinical recurrence after successful CTO recanalization, rendering these difficult procedures more definitive with improved long-term patency. Second, advanced new guidewire techniques have provoked the interest of interventionalists and have increased initial CTO guidewire crossing success. Finally, several innovative technology solutions have been proposed and are being tested which offer the promise of further procedural enhancements, allowing the average interventional operator a greater opportunity for safe and effective CTO therapy.

Considering these dynamic changes in the CTO landscape, it is especially timely to applaud the presentation of this comprehensive *Handbook of Chronic Total Occlusions*. This expertly organized and carefully written handbook represents the collective wisdom of a broad cross-section of CTO treatment experts from around the world. The breadth of topics covered includes general principles of CTO therapy, advanced new guidewire techniques (often pioneered by our Asia-Pacific colleagues), the latest results after drug-eluting stents, and innovative treatment modalities such as radiofrequency ablation, ultrasonic recanalization, excimer laser angioplasty, and blunt dissection techniques. Important areas which address the safety of CTO therapy are also extensively discussed, including specific angiographic and clinical complications during CTO procedures and the more subtle considerations of excessive X-ray exposure and increased radiocontrast volume.

It is particularly noteworthy that this handbook was designed and written specifically for the practicing interventional cardiologist with a special interest in CTO therapy. The content emphasizes operator techniques, clinical treatment issues, and practical case-based scenarios. Undoubtedly, the assimilation of practical materials amassed in this CTO handbook will assist interventional cardiologists in improving their technical skills, and most importantly, the quality of clinical care in patients with complex coronary disease. I heartily recommend this definitive handbook of CTO therapy and expect that it will quickly gain status as a 'must read' text in the subspecialty of interventional cardiology.

Martin B Leon MD
Professor of Medicine
Columbia University Medical Center
New York, NY
USA

Preface

Remarkable progress has been achieved over the past few years in the area of chronic total occlusion (CTO) revascularization. Occurrence of a CTO within a patient's coronary anatomy has been traditionally considered with skepticism from interventional cardiologists. This has been due to the indications and outcomes of percutaneous revascularization as well as the technical difficulties encountered in CTO procedures. Several advances have occurred in all these areas and we had the pleasure to work with a team of worldwide experts in order to present them in a concise and practical way through the present handbook.

The first part of this handbook presents the thought process regarding clinical indications, angiographic stratification of technical difficulty, and the overall planning required before a CTO revascularization in undertaken. The basis interventional concepts of vascular access, guide catheter and wire selection, and manipulation are presented. This part is very critical, since successful wire crossing is the most important step for subsequent equipment passage and a successful procedure. Presentation of these topics extends throughout many chapters, all of which include many case examples with step-by-step explanations of the techniques undertaken. All these three topics are interrelated, since any one of them can ultimately affect wire crossing; all chapters clearly discuss alternative approaches, and corrective pathways and justify the technical options demonstrated in the case examples in a way to promote the necessary synergy among them.

Special attention has been paid to the active support, intravascular ultrasound guidance, and retrograde techniques that have been pioneered by Japanese operators over the past few years. We believe that the careful selection of examples and the painstaking instructions through every single detail of technical principles and related 'tips and tricks' are seminal to CTO procedure teaching.

Following successful crossing, it is still possible that subsequent equipment may not be able to advance through the occlusion. Succeeding in this step is equally important to guidewire crossing of the CTO, and is therefore analyzed at length in this handbook. The instruction provided starts from the importance of vascular access and guide catheter selection, and proceeds to active support techniques (e.g. anchoring balloon) and use of special catheters (e.g. Tornus, excimer laser, etc.), always using telling case examples. The issue of debulking is also presented, including indications and technical suggestions. Finally, the role of drug-eluting stent implantation is presented from two authors in order to best represent the global thought process regarding the long-term procedural outcome.

An operator tackling a CTO lesion needs to be prepared throughout the procedure to deal with certain specific complications. Steps towards avoiding complications by appropriately choosing when to interrupt a CTO procedure (and when to retry later) are discussed in a dedicated chapter. A more rounded review of CTO-specific complications includes many technical details on the ways to manage various types of perforations, as well as the reversal of anticoagulation issues.

Since CTO lesions can also be encountered in the peripheral vascular circulation, we have included dedicated chapters on iliofemoral occlusions, with technical details both on wire crossing as well as on appropriate use of assisting devices (e.g. for distal lumen reentry), again with step-by-step instruction through many selected case examples.

Several 'niche' devices for both coronary and peripheral CTO lesions are presented concisely in dedicated chapters that analyze the current indications, device description, and their technical details utilized in the case demonstrations.

Finally, our general approach for CTO procedure training is outlined with respect to program and individual requirements. Traditionally, training for CTO has been difficult; recent advances can be disseminated though participation in focused courses, preceptorship programs, wider inclusion of CTO in the formal training curriculum, use of simulation, and the work towards building a 'CTO team' of doctors, assisting physicians (trainees) nurses, and technologists within the cardiac catheterization laboratory.

Clearly, we could have expanded each one of the above topics to a much greater length. However, we felt that the concise handbook type of presentation was the most appropriate for the first introduction of this entire subject to the busy interventional cardiology community. We hope that the readers find that we lived up to their expectations.

George D Dangas
Roxana Mehran
Jeffrey W Moses

1

Patient selection and general approach to CTO revascularization

Charles Perry and George D Dangas

Clinical outcomes • Patient selection • General approach • Vascular access • After successful wire crossing

A considerable variety of unsettled issues surround the field of chronic total occlusions (CTOs) as a target for revascularization procedures. There is continual refinement of the following issues: establishment of robust indications, optimal technique, and the ultimate impact of revascularization on patient outcomes. An international expert consensus document has recently addressed these subjects.[1,2] Although other types of revascularization procedures have been established over time based on early results, and then expanded through new indications based on long-term data, this has not been the case for approaching CTO lesions. Difficulty achieving predictable procedural success, together with duration of CTO procedures, (with implications for optimal laboratory time personnel), equipment resource utilization, radiation exposure, and complications, have all posed a unique set of hurdles for routine CTO targeting. Although CTO lesions are observed in approximately one-third of diagnostic coronary arteriograms, recanalization is attempted in less than 15% of patients undergoing percutaneous coronary intervention (PCI).[3,4] Indeed, the most common reason for referral to bypass surgery or exclusion from clinical studies comparing outcomes of angioplasty to bypass surgery has been the presence of a CTO.[5,6]

CLINICAL OUTCOMES

In a large meta-analysis of 4400 patients, Freed et al demonstrated a long-term success rate of 69% in patients after CTO angioplasty, with a major acute cardiovascular event rate of 2%.[7] Long-term success was defined as restriction of lower recurrence of ischemia, improvement of left ventricular function, and higher event-free survival rate. The majority of failures (80%) were free of complications and due to an inability to cross the lesion with a wire, a fact which emphasizes the importance of appropriate patient and material selection. The SICCO trials demonstrated favorable results with stent implantation after successful recanalization; the cardiovascular event rate during 3 years of follow-up was found to be 24% in patients with stents, compared with 59% in conventional angioplasty alone.[8]

The Mid-America Heart Institute Study,[9] British Columbia Cardiac Registry,[10] and Total Occlusion Angioplasty Study (TOAST-GISE)[11] reported on the clinical impact of successful percutaneous CTO revascularization on long-term clinical outcome. The Mid-America Heart Study retrospectively analyzed a consecutive series of 2007 patients over 20 years (1980–1999) of performing PCI for non-acute coronary occlusions. Importantly, long-term survival was similar in patients with successful CTO recanalization compared with a matched cohort of patients undergoing successful angioplasty of non-occluded lesions, and significantly longer than in patients where attempted CTO revascularization failed (10-year survival 74% with CTO success vs 65% with CTO failure; p <0.001). By multivariate analysis, failure to successfully recanalize the CTO was an independent predictor of mortality.

The British Columbia Cardiac Registry studied 1458 patients with CTOs, which constituted 15% of the attempted revascularizations. Successful percutaneous revascularization of CTO was not only associated with increased survival and reduced need for surgical revascularization over 7 years of follow-up but also with a 56% relative reduction in late mortality.

In the prospective TOAST-GISE of 390 CTO (in 369 patients), a successful PCI was associated with: a reduced 12-month incidence of cardiac death or myocardial infarction (1.1% vs 7.2%), a reduced need for coronary artery bypass surgery (2.5% vs 15.7%) and greater freedom from angina (89% vs 75%).

In the overall study population, the only factor associated with enhanced 1-year event-free survival was successful CTO recanalization (odds ratio=0.24; p <0.018).

PATIENT SELECTION

The interventional cardiologist must weigh the individual risks and benefits for each patient when deciding to attempt PCI of a CTO vs two other alternatives: aortocoronary bypass surgery or medical therapy. Clinical, angiographic, and technical considerations must be considered in combination.

From a clinical point of view, age, symptom severity, associated comorbidities (e.g. diabetes mellitus and chronic renal insufficiency), and overall functional status are major determinants of treatment strategy. Angiographically, the extent and complexity of coronary artery disease, likelihood for complete revascularization, and the presence and degree of valvular heart disease and left ventricular dysfunction are all very important factors. The technical probability of achieving successful recanalization of the PCI without complications, as well as the anticipated restenosis rate, must also be heavily weighed in the decision-making process.[2]

When the CTO is the lone obstructive lesion in the coronary vasculature tree, there are three conditions which, when present, favor PCI. The first condition is the presence of symptoms. An average chronic total occlusion with well-developed collaterals is hemodynamically similar to a 90% coronary stenosis without collateral vessels.[12] In a consecutive cohort of 127 patients with visible collaterals and successful CTO recanalization, Werner et al showed that collateral function, measured by intracoronary Doppler and pressure wire indices, was similar in patients with and without post-PCI regional left ventricular functional recovery.[13] Therefore, although considerable recovery of ventricular function after recanalization can be expected (occurring in 39% of patients with baseline ventricular dysfunction in this series), it is independent of invasively determined parameters of collateral function. Coronary collateral development is not closely linked to myocardial viability but is rather the result of the recruitment of preexisting interarterial connections. When successful, the majority of patients with successful CTO recanalization can expect significant reduction or complete resolution of anginal symptoms. In a sample of 10 studies involving 829 patients total, Puma et al found symptom relief is 70% for patients who experienced successful recanalization of the CTO vs only 31% when the attempt was unsuccessful.

The second condition to consider is the presence of viable myocardium. Recovery of left ventricular function in chronically ischemic myocardium depends on the presence of hibernating viable myocardium. In a cohort of 97 patients with CTO, Sirnes et al demonstrated that successful recanalization improved left ventricular ejection fraction by 8.1% (rising from 62% to 67%), with the greatest improvement of 10% occurring in those patients with left anterior descending artery disease.[14] Additionally, they showed that the Wall Motion Severity Index (WMSI), a marker of global left ventricular dysfunction, also increased after CTO recanalization. The WMSI is obtained by averaging the wall motion of all the individual (analyzable) myocardial segments (values: -1 = dyskinesis, 0 = akinesis, 1 = hypokinesis, and 2 = normal).[15] It is notable that the history of MI, the duration of an occlusion, and the incidence of a non-occlusive restenosis had no influence on left ventricular recovery, whereas reocclusion did have an adverse influence.[13]

Finally, the probability of success should steer an operator towards performing PCI in a CTO when the likelihood of success is moderate to high (more than 60%) and the likelihood of complications is low (i.e. anticipated risk of death <1% and MI <5%).[16] Should the PCI attempt prove unsuccessful, further management will depend on the symptomatic status and the extent of jeopardized ischemic myocardium. The operator should therefore be very familiar with the predictors of success when performing PCI of a CTO. Although each condition in Table 1.1 is an independent predictor of success or failure, several factors typically coexist.

Bridging collaterals, which are well-developed vasa vasorum unique to CTO lesions, are proportional to the duration of the CTO and therefore are more common in lesions older than 3 months. If antegrade flow is observed beyond the CTO, it is essential to differentiate the cause as microchannels in the true lumen vs perivascular bridging collaterals: the first is a predictor of success and defines a functional CTO (no longer considered a 'true' CTO), the latter is a predictor of an unsuccessful procedure. The distinction can usually be made by obtaining multiple angiographic projections of the occlusion; however, it sometimes only becomes apparent at the time of PCI. Extensive bridging collaterals that form a 'caput medusae' around the occluded vessel are generally unsuitable for PCI

Table 1.1   Predictors of success and failure in PCI of CTO

Predictors of success	Predictors of failure
Duration <3 months	Duration >3 months
Antegrade flow (+)	Antegrade flow (−)
Tapered morphology (+)	Tapered morphology (−)
Bridging collaterals (−)	Bridging collaterals (+)
Side branch (−)	Side branch (+)
Lesion length <15 mm	Lesion length >15 mm
Single-vessel disease	Multivessel disease

PCI, percutaneous coronary intervention.

due to the very low success rate as well as high complication rate from perforation of the fragile small collateral vessels. However, these classic unfavorable features may no longer constitute unsurpassable hurdles with the employment of the innovative technical approaches described in later chapters of this book. Indeed, several experienced operators consider the absence of a visible distal vessel as the only contraindication to a CTO attempt.

In patients with multivessel disease and one or more CTO lesions, the following conditions suggest careful consideration of referral to bypass surgery in place of attempting PCI: left main stem disease or occluded proximal left anterior descending artery supplying a viable anterior wall, complex triple vessel disease and insulin-requiring diabetes mellitus; severe left ventricular dysfunction; chronic kidney disease. Finally, multiple CTOs with low probability of success or high probability of complication should be treated surgically.

Specifically for patients after a myocardial infarction, two recent trials examined the older concept of "open-artery hypothesis." According to their results,[17-18] sustained potency of an occluded artery can be achieved successfully with percutaneous revascularization. However, in a population that is clinically stable (without significant ischemia of heart failure) and without residual myocardial viability who are submitted to PCI of an occluded artery at least 3 days post-infarction, the revascularization did not seem to confer clinically measurable benefit.

GENERAL APPROACH

Despite the outlined reservations, there has been a gradual increase in technical and procedural success rates for percutaneous CTO recanalization over the last 10 years, as well as an increase in the number of CTO cases attempted. Importantly, this has not been associated with a concomitant increase in adverse event rates, probably related to improved equipment, procedural techniques, operator experience, and improved case selection.[9] Available studies thus far have mostly followed the case-control or cohort methodology. It is difficult to develop prospective, randomized data in the context of an evolving technique and technological approach.

Case selection, angiographic views, and pharmacology

An individualized case selection is of paramount importance for PCI of a CTO. As a general rule, operators should begin with straightforward cases (i.e. patients without any unfavorable features as indicated in Table 1.1) and progressively advance to more complex cases (right column of Table 1.1) as they gain competency. Before performing the procedure, it is essential to review the lesion from multiple views in orthogonal projections. If optimal and detailed visualization is not achieved with conventional angiography, the use of simultaneous ipsilateral and contralateral injections is strongly recommended to define the occluded vessel/stump anatomy, and the presence and orientation of side branches in relation to the assumed true lumen course. It is essential to distinguish microchannels in the CTO lumen, which can be easily perforated and should therefore not be dilated. For the most experienced CTO operator, the only near contraindication to performing percutaneous recanalization of a CTO is the absence of a visible distal vessel lumen (not even through retrograde collaterals).

The amount of contrast load should be thought of prior to the procedure. To economize the amount of contrast used, contralateral injections can be performed through an end-hole catheter inserted distally into the artery for very selective angiography at less than 1 cc per injection. Although this represents the most sensitive approach with respect to contrast media, it may not be advisable routinely due to the risks of a stationary catheter in the distal part of the collateral-providing vessel. For instance, proximal tortuosity and calcification may limit distal positioning or significantly obstruct antegrade flow and increase thrombotic complications.

Since no CTO procedure is considered emergent, appropriate pretreatment with clopidogrel (at least 6 hours prior, but ideally started 3–4 days before at 75 mg daily) and oral aspirin 325 mg should be ensured. Initially, a bolus of 3000 units unfractionated heparin should be administered intravenously or via the guiding catheter; in case contralateral injections will be performed, it is advisable to administer the heparin through the catheter that engages the collateral-providing vessel, especially if a distal indwelling catheter is anticipated. An activated clotting time above 180 seconds is adequate during typical antegrade wire manipulations, but additional heparin may be required for prolonged procedures and particularly if a retrograde approach is followed with advancement of a static catheter system in the collateral-providing vessel; in such cases, a higher activated clotting time is necessary (above 250–300 seconds). When the wire has successfully crossed the lesion and its position in the distal true lumen has been verified, additional heparin should be given to reach an activated clotting time above 250 seconds and a platelet GPIIb/IIIa inhibitor may then be given according to lesion complexity and operator preference. Pharmacological treatment after PCI remains unchanged from the standards applied for PCI performed in non-occlusive stenoses.

VASCULAR ACCESS

Preferred vascular access is usually through the femoral artery, utilizing an 8 Fr guide for passive support, with smaller guides used to provide more maneuverability or for shorter occlusions (in experienced hands). Larger guides, however, provide the ability to introduce covered stents more easily should perforation occur, a possibility that must be entertained for any CTO. If a second catheter is needed for contralateral injections, a 4–6 Fr catheter can be inserted into the opposite femoral artery or either radial artery. Access from the ipsilateral groin using a 4 Fr catheter may also be an acceptable alternative by puncturing 1 cm medially and distally to the previously placed sheath.[19] When a guiding catheter no larger than 6 Fr is required, the distal vessel is visible from ipsilateral collateral flow, and the location of the occlusion is mid or distal in the presence of otherwise favorable anatomy, the radial artery may be an acceptable alternative for CTO angioplasty by experienced radial access operators.[20] If the retrograde approach is entertained, then 8 Fr access should be obtained bilaterally.

Guiding catheter selection

Guiding catheters that provide extra back-up support and coaxial alignment should be chosen. In native coronary arteries, a geometric or left Amplatz guide usually offers the necessary support; however, if a Judkins or Multipurpose is used, the 'deep-seating' maneuver can be employed to achieve the extra back-up. Two guide catheters may be occasionally necessary to image the CTO with contralateral injection, and two 8 Fr guiding catheters are required for the retrograde approach.

For the left coronary system, extra back-up (XB)-type guiding catheters (Voda especially for the circumflex, Extra BackUp especially for the left anterior descending, geometric left, left support) are preferable. Judkins-type guiding catheters provide less support, are associated with reduced success with hard fibrocalcific occlusions, and are not advisable.

For the right coronary artery, left Amplatz 0.75 or 1 (and exceptionally the #2 shape) generally provide the maximal passive support (especially with a superior or shepherd's crook takeoff). On the other hand, acceptable support can be provided in selected cases though hockey-stick shapes for the arteries with transverse or slightly superior takeoffs, or Judkins shapes for inferiorly oriented vessels. Routine use of Judkins, 3-dimensional, or Hockey Stick type catheters may allow better coaxial alignment and wire steerability than Amplatz catheters, and support can be enhanced by special techniques such as the anchoring balloon. In certain cases, coaxial alignment may be more important than passive support (e.g. excessive proximal tortuosity, proximal CTO, unusual location of calcified clefts). Typically, right coronary guiding catheters should have side holes to allow perfusion of the sinus node and conus branches during tight seating of the guide. Aggressive manipulation of the guide catheter, or inadvertent deep intubation (which not infrequently occurs with the Amplatz shape), may dissect the right coronary ostium (often requiring stenting), a complication that should be anticipated and recognized before guidewire removal.

Guidewire selection

This is fundamental for procedural success – the vast majority of failures occur because an operator cannot cross the lesion. Wires designed for treating CTOs can be divided into two groups: polymer-coated (hydrophilic or lubricious) guidewires and non-coated coil guidewires; both groups also possess tapered and non-tapered tips. Operators should become familiar with all wire types, and select certain wires with which to become more comfortable, but still know how to selectively use a significant number of additional wires that are part of the laboratory's 'CTO armamentarium.' Properties of the two wire types are outlined in Table 1.2; other chapters analyze guidewire selection and techniques in detail.

Table 1.2 Characteristics of guidewires for crossing a CTO

Manufacturer	Wire	Shaft and tip diameter	Tip stiffness, (g)	Additional characteristics[a]	Recommended use(s)[b]
Guidant	High torque intermediate	0.014 inch	2–3		1
	High torque standard	0.014 inch	4	a	2, 3
	Cross-It 100	Shaft 0.014 inch Tip 0.010 inch	2	b	1, 4, 10
	Cross-It 200	Shaft 0.014 inch Tip 0.010 inch	3	b	2, 3, 10, 11, 12, 13
	Cross-It 300	Shaft 0.014 inch Tip 0.010 inch	4		
	Cross-It 400	Shaft 0.014 inch Tip 0.010 inch	6	b	5, 8
	Whisper	0.014 inch	1	c, d	1, 4, 6, 7, 9, 10, 13
	Pilot 50	0.014 inch	2	c	1, 4, 6, 7, 9, 10, 13
	Pilot 150 and 200	0.014 inch	4 and 6	e	3, 10, 11, 12, 13
Boston Scientific	Choice PT and P2	0.014 inch	2	d, e, f	1, 4, 6, 7, 9, 10, 13
	PT Graphix and Graphix P2	0.014 inch	3–4	d, e, f	3, 10, 11, 12, 13
	Magnum 0.014	Shaft 0.014 inch Tip 0.7 mm	2	g	1, 13
Asahi Intec	Miracle Brothers	0.014 inch	3, 4, 5, 6, and 12	h, i	1 (3 g), 2, 11 (4.5–6 g), and 2, 5, 8 (12 g); 14 (all)
	Confianza and Confianza Pro (Conquest and Conquest Pro)	Shaft 0.014 inch Tip 0.009 inch	9 and 12	b, i, j, k	2, 5, 8, 10
Johnson and Johnson	Shinobi	0.014 inch	2	c, f, l	9, 10, 11, 13
	Shinobi Plus	0.014 inch	4	c, f, l	2, 3, 9, 10
Terumo	Crosswire EX (platinum) Guidewire GT (gold)	0.016 inch	2	e, m	1, 9, 10

[a]a, caveat: wire entrapment possible in long and hard occlusions; b, tapered tip; c, lubricious tip with non-lubricious shaft; d, difficult to shape tip; e, lubricious shaft and tip; f, poor tip memory; g, olive-shaped ball tip; h, excellent tactile feel; i, excellent torque control within occlusions and in long tortuous lesions; j, Pro version has hydrophilic coating except at distal 1 mm of tip; k, Pro version moves through long occlusions with little resistance; l, caveat: subintimal passage common; m, 45 and 70 degree angles.
[b]1, recent occlusions; 2, chronic occlusions; 3, chronic in-stent occlusions; 4, functional occlusions; 5, long and hard occlusions; 6, subtotal stenoses; 7, acute occlusions; 8, puncturing of fibrous cap; 9, tortuous anatomy; 10, intracoronary microchannels; 11, chronic occlusions <12 months; 12, occluded saphenous vein grafts; 13, recent in-stent occlusions; 14, best for parallel wiring due to excellent torque control. Reproduced from Stone et al,[21] with permission.

AFTER SUCCESSFUL WIRE CROSSING

After passing both the stiff guidewire (non-coated or hydrophilic) and an over-the-wire balloon dilatation catheter through the CTO into the distal lumen, the stiff wire should be immediately withdrawn and replaced with a floppy-tipped non-coated wire to minimize the risk of distal perforation or dissection. Significant problems can arise if the 1.5 mm short balloon cannot be advanced over the wire. This situation calls for additional guide support; since change of a guide catheter over the crossing wire would probably threaten the distal wire position, active support should be attempted using the anchor balloon at a side branch. If this is not effective, an attempt to ablate the lesion with the smallest size (0.7) laser catheter could be attempted, or use of tornus device can be selected. In exceptional cases, the balloon cannot be advanced even over a stiff wire introduced through the tornus. In such cases, it is possible to reinsert the tornus and then exchange the wire for the rota-extra-support and perform rotational atherectomy with the 1.25 burr. All these options are analyzed in dedicated chapters.

After successful dilation of the occlusion, attention must be focused on the entire vessel. Intracoronary administration of nitroglycerin is strongly advised to maximize vasodilation of the chronically underperfused territory. Appropriate predilation should then be performed at all sites that have obstructive lesions, probably including the entire proximal vessel due to the frequently encountered difficulty of advancing long drug-eluting stents through a diseased proximal vessel. If necessary, intravascular ultrasound interrogation may clarify the vessel size and the entire segment length. Finally, drug-eluting stents are recommended to obtain the maximum acute gain and the lowest late loss, since CTO lesions are thought to have exaggerated neointimal proliferative response.[21-23]

At the conclusion of the case, at least one femoral access site can be closed with a device. Closure device choice should be carefully considered if the procedure was unsuccessful and another attempt is planned.

In reviewing several previously attempted CTOs, we have developed the anecdotal observation that a few months of dual antiplatelet therapy can facilitate thrombus resolution and new microchannels can develop after healing of the dissections left at the end of the original procedure that may ultimately facilitate the second attempt. The decision-making process regarding continuation of long CTO procedures vs opting for a future reattempt is discussed in a dedicated chapter.

REFERENCES

1. Stone GW, Reifart NJ, Moussa I, et al. Percutaneous recanalization of chronically occluded coronary arteries: a consensus document: part I. Circulation 2005; 112:2364–72.
2. Stone GW, Reifart NJ, Moussa I, et al. Percutaneous recanalization of chronically occluded coronary arteries: a consensus document: part II. Circulation 2005; 112:2530–7.
3. Anderson HV, Shaw RE, Brindis RG, et al. A contemporary overview of percutaneous coronary interventions. The American College of Cardiology–National Cardiovascular Data Registry (ACC–NCDR). J Am Coll Cardiol 2002; 39(7):1096–103.
4. Srinivas VS, Brooks MM, Detre KM, et al. Contemporary percutaneous coronary intervention versus balloon angioplasty for multivessel coronary artery disease. Circulation 2002; 106(13):1627–33.
5. King SB 3rd, Lembo NJ, Weintraub WS, et al. A randomized trial comparing coronary angioplasty with coronary bypass surgery. N Engl J Med 1994; 331:1044–50.

6. Bourassa MG, Roubin GS, Detre KM, et al. Bypass Angioplasty Revascularization Investigation: patient screening, selection, and recruitment. Am J Cardiol 1995; 75:3C–8C.
7. Freed J, et al. Meta-analysis of chronic total occlusion PTCA outcome. In: Chevalier B, Royer T, Guyton Ph, Glatt B, eds. Chronic Total Occlusions. Paris Course on Revascularization 2001, Marco J, ed, Europa edition, Paris 2001:127–42.
8. Sirnes PA, Golf S, Myreng Y, et al. Stenting in Chronic Coronary Occlusion (SICCO): a randomized, controlled trial of adding stent implantation after successful angioplasty. J Am Coll Cardiol 1996; 28(6):1444–51.
9. Suero JA, Marso SP, Jones PG, et al. Procedural outcomes and long-term survival among patients undergoing percutaneous coronary intervention of a chronic total occlusion in native coronary arteries: a 20-year experience. J Am Coll Cardiol 2001; 38:409–14.
10. Ramanathan K, Gao M, Nogareda GJ, et al. Successful percutaneous recanalization of a non-acute occluded coronary artery predicts clinical outcomes and survival. Circulation, 2001; 104:II-415.
11. Olivari Z, Rubartelli P, Piscione F, et al. for the TOAST-GISE Investigators: data from a multicenter, prospective, observational study (TOASTGISE). J Am Coll Cardiol 2003; 41:1672–8.
12. Flameng W, Schwarz F, Hehrlein FW, et al. Intraoperative evaluation of the functional significance of coronary collateral vessels in patients with coronary artery disease. Am J Cardiol 1978; 42:187–92.
13. Werner GS, Surber R, Kuethe F, et al. Collaterals and the recovery of left ventricular function after recanalization of a chronic total coronary occlusion. Am Heart J 2005; 149(1):129–37.
14. Sirnes PA, Myreng Y, Molstad P, Bonarjee V, Golf S. Improvement of left ventricular ejection fraction and wall motion after successful recanalization of chronic coronary occlusions. Eur Heart J 1998; 19:273–81.
15. Jensen-Urstad K, Bouvier F, Hojer J, et al. Comparison of different echocardiographic methods with radionuclide imaging for measuring left ventricular ejection fraction during acute myocardial infarction treated by thrombolytic therapy. Am J Cardiol 1998; 81:538–44.
16. Kereiakes DJ, Selmon MR, McAuley BJ, et al. Angioplasty in total coronary artery occlusion: experience in 76 consecutive patients. J Am Coll Cardiol 1985; 6:526–33.
17. Hochman Is, Lamas GA, Buller CE, et al. Coronary intervention for persistent occlusion after myocardial infarction. N Engl J Med 2006; 355:2395–2407.
18. Dzavik V, Buller CE, Lamas GA, et al. Randomized trial of percutaneous coronary interventions for subacute inarct related coronary occlusion to achieve long-term patency and improve ventricular function: the Total Occlusion Study of Canada (TOSCA) – 2 trial. Circulation 2006; 114:2449–2457.
19. Reifart N. Contralateral injections for chronic total occlusions using 4 F and the same groin. In: Katoh O, Margolis J, Reifart N, Virmani R, eds. Chronic Total Occlusion Pathophysiology, Intervention and Expert Case Management. Santa Clara, CA: Guidant Publications; 2001: 16–31.
20. Kiemeneij F, Laarman GJ, de Melker E. Transradial artery coronary angioplasty. Am Heart J 1995; 129:1–7.
21. Suttorp et al. for the PRISON II Investigators. Prospective Randomized Trial of Sirolimus-Eluting and Bare Metal Stents in Patients With Chronic Total Occlusions (PRISON II). Results presented at TCT 2005, Washington, DC.
22. Buller CE, Dzavik V, Carere RG, et al. Primary stenting versus balloon angioplasty in occluded coronary arteries: the Total Occlusion Study of Canada (TOSCA). Circulation 1999; 100(3):236–42.
23. Stone GW, Colombo A, Teirstein PS, et al. Percutaneous recanalization of chronically occluded coronary arteries: procedural techniques, devices, and results. Catheter Cardiovasc Interv 2005; 66:217–36.

2

Guidewire techniques and technologies: hydrophilic versus stiff wire selection

Garrett B Wong, Matthew J Price, and Paul S Teirstein

Lesion characteristics • Guidewire selection • Conclusion

Chronic total occlusion (CTO) remains one of the most difficult challenges for the interventional cardiologist. Both short- and long-term outcomes of patients with CTOs are related to procedural success.[1-6] Recent advancements in guidewire technology have improved the technical success of approaching difficult CTOs, such as occlusions that are calcified, long, and/or old. Success rates that were historically 50–70%[7,8] have now improved, for many interventionalists, to 80–90%.

Guidewires are available in a large variety of lengths, tip diameters and shapes, coatings, stiffnesses, and materials. Guidewires can be classified into several dichotomous categories: hydrophilic vs hydrophobic, stiff vs soft, supportive vs non-supportive, and tapered vs non-tapered. This chapter focuses, on guidewire technology and the appropriate selection of wires for different subsets of chronic occlusions.

LESION CHARACTERISTICS

The overall success rate of opening CTOs depends on several lesion-specific characteristics, which affects the selection of the appropriate guidewire. Known predictors of success are:

- the duration that the vessel has been closed
- the length of the occlusion
- the presence or absence of antegrade flow
- the presence or absence of a stump
- the presence or absence of bridging collaterals.[8-10]

Collateralization of the distal vessel demonstrating a 'target' for guidewire passage can impact the success rate of crossing and ultimately recanalizing the occluded vessel. There are multiple types of neovascularization, which may develop in the setting of a highly stenosed lesion. Both ipsilateral and contralateral collaterals may develop. Ipsilateral collaterals may be either epicardial angiographic bridging collaterals or true microvascular collaterals. The particular type of neovascular development often dictates the type of guidewire that is used to cross the lesion.

Plaque composition is another important factor in the success or failure of CTO revascularization. Histopathological evaluation of various lesions has allowed the characterization of plaques, which can be roughly classified as 'soft', 'hard', or a combination of both.[11] Hard plaques are more prevalent in CTO lesions with increasing age. A dense fibrotic lesion may not be crossed with a typical workhorse wire and ultimately may require a stiffer guidewire to 'push' through the hard plaque. In addition, calcification within the plaque adds a level of complexity to the percutaneous coronary intervention (PCI) procedure. The fibrocalcific segments of the plaque are more likely to deflect the guidewire tip and lead to subintimal dissections and possibly perforations.

GUIDEWIRE SELECTION

Hydrophilic guidewires

Hydrophilic guidewires have special coatings engineered from absorbent materials, which become slippery upon contact with liquids, such as saline or blood. There are various polymeric coatings currently being utilized by the guidewire manufacturers to optimize wire performance and affect the degree of hydrophilicity. The chemical properties of these polymeric coatings create a lubricious surface that allows the guidewire to slide through tortuous segments and small channels easier than a non-hydrophilic wire. The hydrophilic-coated guidewires are typically useful in lesions which have visible channels that allow the wire to navigate through the stenosed segment or segments. Additionally, these wires are superior for markedly tortuous vessels and lesions, allowing the wire to glide through and conform to the highly stenosed regions and around tight bends with more ease. The wires are designed to offer little resistance when they contact the vessel wall and soft tissue. The operator must therefore be cautious with the polymer-coated wires as they can easily find there way into a false lumen with less tactile feedback, which, if not recognized, can lead to significant intimal dissection and procedural failure. In rare cases, this can cause coronary perforation and subsequent cardiac tamponade.

There are a multitude of hydrophilic guidewires currently available, including the Abbott Vascular (previously Guidant) Whisper and Hi-Torque Pilot series, Asahi Intec Confianza Pro, Boston Scientific Choice PT and PT Graphix, Cordis Shinobi and Shinobi Plus, and the Terumo Crosswire. The wires have a broad range of torque response and lateral stiffness characteristics. In the setting of a chronic occlusion, these slippery wires can be very useful in finding microchannels through the difficult or tortuous lesion. In addition, once the lesion is successfully crossed, the hydrophilic wires will easily track through the often small and underfilled distal vessel with ease. Compared with non-hydrophilic wires, hydrophilic wires excel in moving through occluded and calcified vessels but, as a class, are generally less steerable than non-hydrophilic wires.

Hydrophilic guidewires have been compared with conventional wires in small series of coronary intervention procedures. In a study by Lefèvre and colleagues,[12] conventional non-coated wires were compared with the Terumo Crosswire for difficult-to-cross lesions. When the hydrophilic Crosswire was used as the initial guidewire, the success rate in crossing the lesion was 74% vs 35% for the conventional wire (Table 2.1). When a conventional wire failed as the initial approach, which occurred in 59% of the patients, more than a third of the lesions were successfully traversed when crossed-over to the hydrophilic wire. In addition, a significant decrease in number of guidewires used and the overall procedure time were seen with the hydrophilic Crosswire.

Calcific or densely fibrotic lesions can be difficult to cross with the hydrophilic coated guidewires. Several wires are available in different stiffnesses, such as the Abbott Vascular Hi-Torque Pilot family, which includes wires with increasing tip stiffness from the 50, to the 150, and up to the 200 (Figure 2.1). The increased tip stiffness translates into more torque transmission and tip control (Figure 2.2). All of these guidewires have a proprietary polymer coating to increase the hydrophilicity. The stiffer, more powerful hydrophilic wires may allow the penetration of the lesion cap, but this property may be disadvantageous in certain lesion subsets. The calcified or thick fibrotic cap of certain total occlusions may deflect the tip of these slick, stiff guidewires into a subintimal plane or through the vessel wall, leading to a dissection or, rarely, to a perforation. Therefore, it is important to emphasize the importance of visualization of the distal vessel via ipsilateral or contralateral collaterals when using these wires. The use of multiple, orthogonal views can be very useful to determine whether or not the distal wire is truly in the proper vessel lumen. The lubricious coatings on these types of wires can almost effortlessly allow the wires to continue to propagate extraluminally alongside the true lumen once a false channel has been entered, especially with the stiffer wires. Guidewire positioning should certainly be verified before any balloon inflations are performed. A useful technique is to employ the Dotter method,[13] simply passing a balloon catheter in and out through the lesion prior to any balloon inflations, which can often discern whether or not the appropriate pathway has been taken with the wire. If there is any evidence of extraluminal staining consistent with a dissection, the wire can be withdrawn and redirected until the true lumen is found. Distal balloon injection with contrast can also be useful to verify wire position, but does not guarantee that the wire remains intraluminal for the entire course, and in some cases the contrast injection may propagate the dissection plane laterally and distally. Once the proper distal wire position is secured, the

Table 2.1   Conventional guidewire compared with the Terumo Crosswire

Parameter	Conventional (n = 46)	Crosswire (n = 42)	p value
First guidewire success (%)	35	74	0.001
Crossover (%)	59	26	0.009
Guidewire success after crossover (%)	37	0	<0.001
Total guidewire number	1.7 ± 0.6	1.3 ± 0.5	<0.001
Procedure (min)	84 ± 33	42 ± 20	0.013

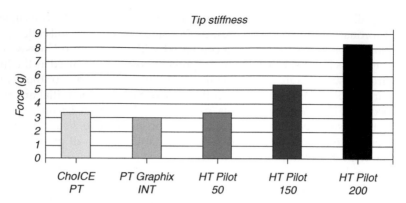

Figure 2.1   Comparison of guidewire tip stiffness.

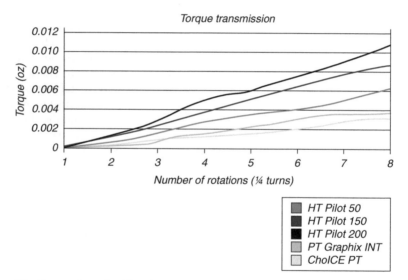

Figure 2.2   Comparison of guide wire torque transmission.

hydrophilic wire should be exchanged for a less traumatic and/or more supportive wire to facilitate the angioplasty and stenting of the vessel and prevent distal dissection or perforation by the hydrophilic wire during stent manipulation.

Certain lesion subsets do not favor an initial hydrophilic guidewire approach. A heavily fibrotic or calcific lesion cap may not be crossable with a polymer-coated wire. Likewise, a flush occlusion at a side branch is highly unfavorable as the lubricious guidewire will have a tendency to deflect off of the lesion and track into the side branch. In these settings, the operator must exercise great care in wire management so as to not complicate the case any further with a wire dissection or perforation. These lesions typically will require the use of the stiffer, non-hydrophilic group of wires.

One recently described technique using hydrophilic guidewires is to use their lubricity to intentionally enter a false channel, form a J loop in the guidewire, and use a support catheter to push the loop distally through the vessel wall until it breaks through to the true lumen. This technique has been called the STAR (subintimal tracking and reentry) technique and has been more successful in chronic right coronary occlusions which typically have the major side branches located distally, as described in detail in Chapter 5.[14]

Another recently introduced approach is to take advantage of the collateral circulation to perform a retrograde recanalization.[15] Typically, septal collaterals are used to pass from the right posterior descending artery (PDA) to the left anterior descending artery (LAD) or from the LAD to the PDA. A hydrophilic guidewire is used with a very low profile over-the-wire balloon catheter or hydrophilic-coated support catheter. This technique is quite new and its success, failure, and complication rates have not yet been well defined; a dedicated chapter analyzes this technical approach.

Stiff guidewires

Stiff guidewires make up the remainder of the coronary guidewires for approaching CTOs. These wires have a standard, non-hydrophilic coil tip designed to facilitate the penetration of either the proximal or distal cap, especially when the cap is fibrotic and hard. In contrast to the typical workhorse wire with relatively floppy tips and mild to moderate body support, these wires are designed to allow sufficient transmission of steerability and crossing force at the target lesion.

The newest generation of more supportive, stiffer hydrophobic guidewires includes the Asahi Intec Miraclebros series, and the tapered tip wires such as the Asahi Intec Confianza and Abbott Vascular Hi-Torque Cross-It. These wires offer superior torquability and tactile 'feel' for the lesions. The Asahi Intec guidewires have a one-piece wire core that provides accurate 1:1 torque response, pushability, and steerability. These wires vary in tip stiffness from the Miraclebros 3g (3 tip load), 4.5g, 6g, and up to the Miraclebros 12g. As the tip stiffness increases, the torque transmission improves, with the tradeoff of less tip resistance transmission for the operator. The Confianza series (also known as the Conquest outside the USA) has a tapered tip from 0.014 inch down to 0.009 inch and carries either a 9g or 12g tip load. The tapered segment provides greater penetration force and less tip resistance than non-tapered wires. The Confianza Pro is a hybrid wire which has a hydrophilic coating on all but its distal non-hydrophilic tip to allow improved torquability and passage through fibrocalcific obstructions while minimizing the risk of entering a false channel. The non-tapered Miraclebros family of wires offer better torque performance and tactile feel, but less penetration force than the Confianza family. The Abbott Vascular Hi-Torque Cross-It wires have a similar tapered tip from 0.014 inch to 0.010 inch over the last 3 cm, but these wires also have a hydrophilic coating over the tapered segment to allow smoother tracking and enhance the crossing capabilities. This series of wires is available with increasing stiffness from the Cross-It 100 to the Cross-It 200, 300, and 400 guidewires.

Tapered-tip guidewires have been shown to provide a significant benefit in overall success rate of CTO PCI compared with conventional guidewires.[16]

In this retrospective study, 182 patients underwent PCI for CTO lesions of >3-month duration. There were no significant differences in clinical or lesion characteristics except for the use of tapered-tip guidewires. The overall success rate of PCI was improved significantly with the use of tapered-tip guidewires, specifically in tapered-type occlusions ($p = 0.002$) and shorter lengths of occlusion ($p = 0.004$).

These newer generations of stiff wires excel in the chronic occlusions that have known unfavorable characteristics: thickened, fibrotic proximal and distal caps, convex lesions with no distal tapering, relatively long lesions, and occlusions that terminate at a significant side branch. These wires offer pushability through the lesion with excellent tip control and torque response. Therefore, the operator can steer away from the side branch or enter a lesion cap with the necessary control to minimize complications. However, in a tortuous segment of the lesion, the wire stiffness makes it more challenging to follow the true pathway beyond a sharp turn, which can result in a subintimal dissection. The parallel wire technique can be useful in this setting to attempt to cross through the lesion into the true distal lumen. In this situation, the initial guidewire is left in the false channel when reentry into the true lumen cannot be accomplished. A second guidewire, typically with a different tip shape or stiffness, is then inserted alongside, or parallel, to the initial wire. The goal is to advance the additional wire into the distal lumen beyond the occlusion and to not continue reentering the subintimal space created by the first wire. Our experience has demonstrated that a stiff, non-hydrophilic guidewire is the preferred wire to optimize this technique.

Algorithm for guidewire selection

When approaching CTOs, the selection of the appropriate guidewire is critical to the ultimate success or failure of the procedure. The operator must tailor the particular wire to the specific lesion characteristics, as there is, unfortunately, not a single wire that will be suitable for every CTO lesion subset. Wire exchanges during the course of the procedure are common as the intervention progresses, as the need for different wire characteristics dictates. Lesion chronicity, if known, plays a role in the guidewire selection process. More recent occlusions are typically less fibrotic than much older occlusions and may be crossed relatively easily without the need for significant pushability.

An effective method of guidewire selection is to use a gradual step-up approach (Figure 2.3). At our center, we will typically probe the lesion initially with a standard workhorse wire (e.g. Abbott Vascular Balanced Middleweight or Asahi Prowater) loaded in an over-the-wire balloon or other type of support catheter to facilitate wire exchanges. Occasionally one is surprised by the ease of lesion crossing. If there is any resistance at the lesion and there are no visible angiographic microchannels conducive to the use of a hydrophilic wire, we routinely exchange for our initial CTO guidewire, which is usually the Miraclebros 3 (MB3). Guidewire shaping is an important factor, as a smaller curve on the wire tip is favorable to a large curve to allow more coaxial force transmission at the lesion. In harder, more fibrotic lesions, the MB3 may not offer the penetration force to cross the lesion cap. A stepwise approach is to use the Miraclebros 4.5, then the Miraclebros 6, and then ultimately advancing to the Miraclebros 12 or switching to the Confianza series or Cross-It series. By gradually choosing stiffer wires with

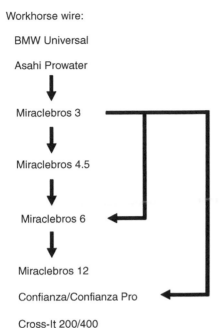

Workhorse wire:

BMW Universal

Asahi Prowater

Miraclebros 3

Miraclebros 4.5

Miraclebros 6

Miraclebros 12

Confianza/Confianza Pro

Cross-It 200/400

Figure 2.3 Guidewire selection – step-up approach.

higher tip loads, one can select the wire with the sufficient crossing force to successfully penetrate the lesion (while minimizing the chance of vessel perforation with an overly stiff wire) while maximizing the feel of the wire response. As the tip stiffness increases, however, the tactile feel of the guidewires decreases. Once the lesion has been successfully crossed, the stiff wire should be exchanged out for a standard workhorse wire with a standard curve on the wire tip. Occasionally a more supportive wire may be required to deliver the appropriate equipment through the total occlusion.

An alternative approach is to again get an initial feel for the lesion with the MB3 wire, but then move directly to a very stiff wire or a tapered tip wire if the lesion appears to have a hard cap. This approach may be appropriate in very old occlusions, which have a tendency to being more fibrotic, and possibly calcified. The very stiff Miraclebros 12, the tapered tip Confianza wires, particularly the Confianza Pro, Confianza Pro 12, and the Cross-It 200, 300, or 400, are the wires of choice when in this situation. This is our preferred approach, in particular for the lesion that is rather short with good distal collateralization but has a hard, fibrous cap. In this situation, pushability and penetrability are the main requirements for success. The difficult CTO with the flush occlusion at a significant side branch is also better suited for these stiffer, non-hydrophilic guidewires. A hydrophilic guidewire in this situation will have a tendency to select the side branch rather than penetrate the proximal lesion cap. The stiffer, non-coated wire tips will minimize the deflection off of the hard lesion into the side branches.

During the course of a given PCI procedure of a CTO, the operator is often faced with multiple complex decisions. For example, the initial portion of the lesion may be quite tortuous and subtotally occluded for a significant length of vessel, at which point the vessel becomes a total flush occlusion at the takeoff of a sizeable side branch. This specific scenario may require multiple types of guidewires to successfully negotiate the vessel. Again, an over-the-wire balloon catheter or other support catheter will allow the operator to easily switch wires, depending on the demands of the vessel segment. A hydrophilic steerable guidewire would be the initial wire of choice for the tortuous, tiny channel to navigate through the lengthy proximal segment. However, once the CTO at the takeoff of a side branch is reached, a non-hydrophilic, stiff and powerful guidewire with a tapered tip may be utilized to cross the fibrous cap of the true total occlusion, often in a stepwise approach with progressively stiffer wires. It is important to know the strengths and limitations of the various wires, and one should be careful not to attempt to force a particular wire to open a CTO that may not be amenable to the characteristics of that given wire. Occasionally, a given CTO may be 'partially' opened despite the inability to completely access the distal true lumen. In such cases, recanalization may be reattempted a few weeks later; the lesion may now demonstrate a small channel, simplifying the procedure substantially.

CONCLUSION

Chronic total occlusions represent one of the most difficult procedural challenges for interventional cardiologists. Previous lesion subsets that were once thought to be untreatable by percutaneous intervention are now being successfully opened as physician experience and guidewire innovations continue to improve. An individualized lesion-based approach is necessary when treating chronic coronary occlusions, because the anatomy of total occlusions varies. Proper knowledge of the advantages and limitations of the different guidewires, in particular the nuances between hydrophilic and stiffer guidewires, is essential to improving the likelihood of procedural success. The operator should not hesitate to change guidewires and strategies throughout the course of the intervention as the case progresses in order to utilize the strengths of each wire. In the future, with increasing experience and evolutionary advances in guidewire technology, the final frontier of percutaneous revascularization – the chronic total occlusion – may be conquered.

REFERENCE

1. Suero JA, Marso SP, Jones PG, et al. Procedural outcome and long term survival among patients undergoing percutaneous coronary intervention of a chronic total occlusion in native coronary arteries: a 20 year experience. J Am Coll Cardiol 2001; 38(2):409–14.
2. Choi SW, Lee CW, Hong MK, et al. Clinical and angiographic follow-up after long versus short stenting in unselected chronic coronary occlusions. Clin Cardiol 2003; 26:265–8.
3. Rubartelli P, Verna E, Niccoli L, et al. Gruppo Italiano di Studio sullo Stent nelle Occlusioni Coronariche Investigators. Coronary stent implantation is superior to balloon angioplasty for chronic coronary occlusions: six-year clinical follow-up of the GISSOC trial. J Am Coll Cardiol 2003; 41:1488–92.
4. Hoye A, Tanabe K, Lemos PA, et al. Significant reduction in restenosis after the use of sirolimus-eluting stents in the treatment of chronic total occlusions. J Am Coll Cardiol 2004; 43:1954–8.
5. Werner GS, Krack A, Schwarz G, et al. Prevention of lesion recurrence in chronic total occlusions by paclitaxel-eluting stents. J Am Coll Cardiol 2004; 44:23301–6.

6. Ge L, Iakovou I, Cosgrave J, et al. Immediate and mid-term outcomes of sirolimus-eluting stent implantation for chronic total occlusions. Eur Heart J 2005; 26:1049–51.

7. Hoye A, van Domburg RT, Sonnenschein K, Serruys PW. Percutaneous coronary intervention for chronic total occlusions: the thoraxcenter experience 1992–2002. Eur Heart J 2005; 26: 2630–6.

8. Stone GW, Rutherford BD, McConahay DR, et al. Procedural outcome of angioplasty for total coronary artery occlusion: an analysis of 971 lesions in 905 patients. J Am Coll Cardiol 1990; 15:849–56.

9. Tan KH, Sulke N, Taub NA, et al. Determinants of success of coronary angioplasty in patients with a chronic total occlusion: a multiple logistic regression model to improve selection of patients. Br Heart 1993; 70:126–31.

10. Dong S, Smorgick Y, Nahir M, et al. Predictors for successful angioplasty of chronic totally occluded coronary arteries. J Interv Cardiol 2005; 18:1–7.

11. Stone GW, Kandzari DE, Mehran R, et al. Percutaneous recanalization of chronically occluded coronary arteries: a consensus document: part I. Circulation 2005; 112:2364–72.

12. Lefèvre T, Louvard Y, Loubeyre C, et al. A randomized study comparing two guidewire strategies for angioplasty of chronic total coronary occlusion. Am J Cardiol 2000; 85:1144–7.

13. Dotter CT, Rosch J, Judkins MP. Transluminal dilatation of atherosclerotic stenosis. Surg Gynecol Obstet 1968; 127:794–804.

14. Colombo A, Mikhail GW, Michev I, et al. Treating chronic total occlusions using subintimal tracking and reentry: the STAR technique. Catheter Cardiovasc Interv 2005; 64:407–11.

15. Rosenmann D, Meerkin D, Almagor Y. Retrograde dilatation of chronic total occlusions via collateral vessel in three patients. Catheter Cardiovasc Interv 2006; 67:250–3.

16. Saito S, Tanaka S, Hiroe Y, et al. Angioplasty for chronic total occlusion by using tapered-tip guidewires. Catheter Cardiovasc Interv 2003; 59:305–11.

3

Advanced techniques for antegrade advancement of wires

Etsuo Tsuchikane

Parallel wiring technique • Seesaw wiring technique • Anchoring balloon technique • IVUS guidance • Conclusions

The antegrade advancement of wires through a chronic total occlusion (CTO) is not only dependent on the type of wires used but also on the utilization of several special techniques that can enhance procedural success. In order to be able to take advantage of these techniques, the interventionist needs to understand their technical details in a very organized fashion.

PARALLEL WIRING TECHNIQUE

This technique is the most important in the current wiring techniques for CTO. Usually we start to tackle the CTO by single wire manipulation under fluoroscopy. However, sometimes this first wire slips into a subintimal space despite careful wire handling. This is a common, usual situation in percutaneous coronary intervention (PCI) of CTO. The important thing is to understand the ramifications of the next step. In these situations, operators tend to pull back and push the same wire to seek the true channel. However, this procedure easily creates expansion of the subintimal space, leading to true channel collapse, which in turn makes it more difficult to recanalize the true lumen. Furthermore, to check the position of the wire tip during single-wire manipulation, contrast media injections are conducted frequently (both in fluoroscopy and in cineangiographic modes), leading to increased radiation and contrast exposure. It is notable that forceful antegrade injections also cause expansion of the subintimal space.

Therefore, once the first wire enters into the subintimal space, one may try to get to the true channel by manipulating this wire's course intentionally; however, this should be tried only a few times and one should never move this wire any more unless those reattempts are successful.

The first wire should be left in place, and then a second wire should be delivered under the guidance (landmark) of the first wire, which usually indicates the correct position of the true channel (Figure 3.1). The second wire should follow a course according to the lessons learned from the first wire's failure. The concept

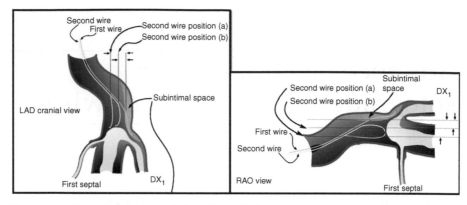

Figure 3.1 The concept of parallel wiring technique. This is a scheme of parallel wiring technique in an LAD CTO (left anterior descending artery chronic total occlusion) case. The first wire is slipping into the subintimal space in the pericardial side. To prevent the further expansion of subintimal space, the first wire must be left there as an indicator for the second wire. The second wire should be carefully advanced towards the distal end, so that it is positioned between (a) and (b). Finally, the distal fibrous cap should be penetrated from this position by using a stiffer wire than the first wire. RAO, right anterior oblique; DX_1 first diagonal branch.

of parallel wiring technique also includes the saving of multiple antegrade contrast injections and avoidance of further expansion of subintimal space, since the first wire serves as a landmark.

In order to change the wire course intentionally, the second wire usually has a stiffer tip wire than the first wire. Depending on the lesion morphology, one may use a tapered stiff wire such as the Confianza (Asahi Intec, Japan) in a short and straight CTO to change the course and penetrate the distal fibrous cap (Figure 3.2). Nonetheless, one should also consider a stiff wire with better torque performance such as the Miraclebros (Asahi Intec, Japan) family when trying to negotiate a CTO in a tortuous vessel (Figure 3.3). Hydrophilic-coating stiff tip wires cannot be recommended in the parallel wiring technique because they tend to slip into the subintimal space.

Since a support catheter is required for wire handling in PCI of CTO, the operator has to retrieve the support catheter from the first wire and then deliver it again with the second wire when using a small size of guiding catheter (6 Fr). When using a big size of guiding catheter (7 or 8 Fr), a second support system can be inserted for the second wire without retrieval of the initial support system. In such cases, one can easily move on to the seesaw wiring technique, as mentioned below. We usually use a big size of guiding catheter (8 Fr) in PCI of CTO so that we can use any kind of wiring technique in addition to enhanced back-up force. To have a greater chance of achieving successful recanalization, one should prepare with all the favorable conditions from the beginning of the procedure; accordingly, we usually employ an 8 Fr guiding catheter system.

SEESAW WIRING TECHNIQUE

The seesaw wiring technique, another type of parallel wiring technique, should be called an 'alternative parallel wiring'. This technique requires two support

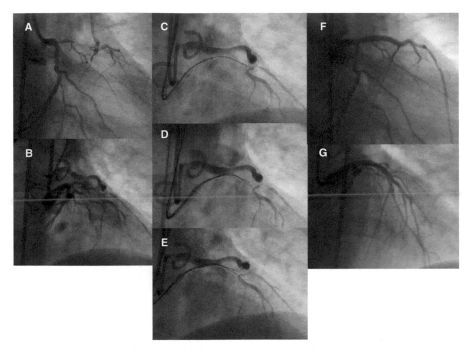

Figure 3.2 Case example of an LAD CTO (left anterior descending artery chronic total occlusion). A middle-aged male patient with bypass graft failure to the LAD area. The proximal LAD was almost straight and the occlusion length was not so long (A, B). After the first wire (Miraclebros 6) entered into the subintimal space (C), the second wire (Confianza) was easily and successfully led into the distal true channel under the marker of the first wire (D, E). Final angiographic result after stenting (F, G). In these cases with a short occlusion in the non-tortuous vessel, a tapered stiff wire is easily controlled.

catheter systems. When the second wire also slips into the subintimal space in the parallel wiring technique, it is used as a new indicator. Then the first wire should be retrieved from the support catheter and another stiff wire (same as or stiffer than the second wire) is delivered to negotiate the lesion. The operator can move these two wire systems alternatively when necessary; this procedure is called the 'seesaw wiring technique'. This technique has a high risk of worsening the subintimal dilatation and may further compress the true lumen compared with the basic 'parallel wire' technique. Therefore, routine use of this technique cannot be recommended; if it is used, more careful wire handling is mandatory.

ANCHORING BALLOON TECHNIQUE

When the wire is unable to be advanced in the hard CTO lesion, the guiding catheter and/or the support microcatheter necessarily gets pushed back during wire handling. The unstable back-up condition prohibits appropriate wire manipulation and may lead to complete equipment dislodgement from the target artery in case it is not attended to properly. The anchoring balloon technique is an effective alternative for these situations. Two methods employ this technique.

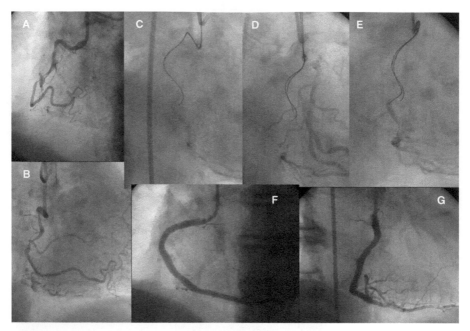

Figure 3.3 Case example of an RCA CTO (right coronary artery chronic total occlusion). An advanced-age female patient with post-infarction angina. Although the occlusion length was not long, the RCA vessel was tortuous (A, B). The first wire, Miraclebros 3, delivered to negotiate the occlusion slipped into the subintimal space (C). Then the second wire, Miraclebros 6, was carefully advanced using the parallel wiring technique (D) and a successful wire crossing was achieved (E). Final angiographic result after stenting (F, G). In a CTO located in a tortuous vessel, wires with high-torque performance should be used, particularly for the second wire in the parallel wiring technique.

The first method aims to stabilize the guiding catheter and is useful in the treatment of proximal CTO, particularly in right coronary cases (Figure 3.4). In such situations, positioning and inflating a balloon in the conus branch or in an acute marginal makes the guiding catheter stabilized, as an anchor. The size of balloon should be matched to the size of the branch: a little bit bigger but inflated at low pressure is the best combination in my experience. This procedure has a risk of sinus bradycardia when the balloon is inflated in the conus branch. This complication actually occurs rarely, and can be dealt with by conducting intermittent inflations. Since two catheter systems are needed for this technique, an 8 Fr guiding catheter is again preferable.

The second method is to use an inflated over-the-wire (OTW) balloon during wire handling. When a tight proximal fibrous cap cannot be penetrated, one can enforce the back-up support by inserting and inflating a balloon over the working wire (Figure 3.5). In addition, the guiding catheter can be engaged deeply by pulling on the inflated anchor balloon system. The size of the OTW balloon should be matched to the reference lumen size proximal to the CTO. When a long occluded CTO is attempted, a 1.5 OTW balloon can be used for this purpose by inflating it inside the CTO. However, one should be careful not to dilate the

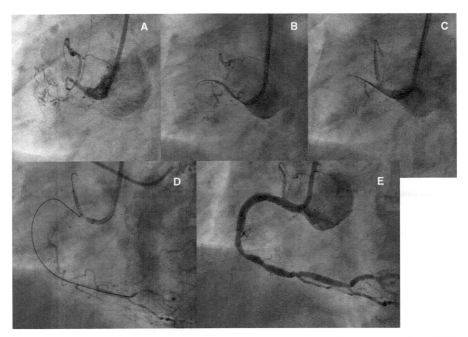

Figure 3.4 Case example of an RCA CTO (right coronary artery chronic total occlusion). A middle-aged male patient with stable angina. The proximal RCA was completely blocked with bridging collaterals (A). To prevent damage to the RCA ostium by the guiding catheter, a Judkins-type catheter was used. However, because of the tight plaque in the CTO, the guiding catheter was unstable during the wire handling so that the wire could not be advanced intentionally (B). Then, a 2.5 mm balloon was inserted and inflated with a low pressure in the conus branch to stabilize the guiding catheter (C). Under the use of this anchoring balloon, the wire control was improved, so that the occlusion was successfully negotiated (D). Final angiographic result after stenting (E).

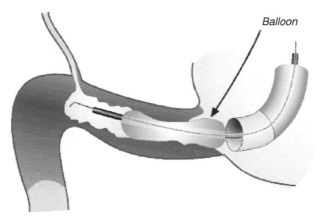

Balloon

Figure 3.5 Another kind of anchoring balloon technique. This is a scheme of another type of anchoring technique by using an over-the-wire (OTW) balloon. When the proximal fibrous cap cannot be penetrated even by using a stiff wire, an OTW balloon may be dilated proximal to the occlusion as a support catheter. The inflated balloon makes an extra back-up force for the wire tip to break down the proximal cap.

false channel in the CTO. This technique may be particularly helpful for targeting long CTO lesions that have several 'islands;' The 1.5 OTW balloon can be dilated inside the first island with a certainty of being intraluminal, and proceeds superior back-up support when manipulating the wire towards subsequent 'islands' through the CTO.

IVUS GUIDANCE

Intravascular ultrasound (IVUS) sometimes plays an important role for procedural success of CTO, because it can provide us with the cross-sectional morphology and size information that we cannot obtain with fluoroscopy. During wire handling for CTO, IVUS could be effective for two settings: one is to confirm the entrance of the CTO and the other to penetrate from the false to the true channel.

When there is no stump at the entrance of the CTO, an entry point may not be located. In such cases, IVUS can locate the beginning of the CTO with certainty (Figure 3.6). In a similar situation, even when we can easily identify the entrance,

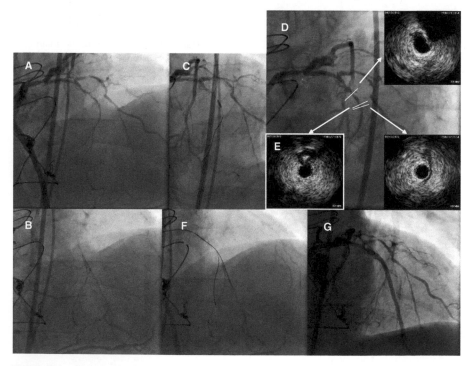

Figure 3.6 Case example of an LAD CTO (left anterior descending artery chronic total occlusion). A middle-aged male patient with angina. Although the LAD was completely blocked around the mid portion, it was hard to identify the entrance to the CTO, even when the contralateral injection was performed (A, B). Then, an IVUS catheter was inserted into the septal branch (C) so that the IVUS image easily indicated the CTO entrance (D, E). This confirmation also facilitated the aggressive use of a stiff wire to penetrate the proximal cap (F). Final angiographic result after stenting (G).

it is sometimes important to check the entry point of the wire very early in the procedure, because the wire may easily enter the subintimal space from the wrong entry point in a CTO without stump. A case example is shown in Figure 3.7. It is recommended that when you meet a CTO without a stump but a side branch big enough to deliver an IVUS catheter, one should consider using IVUS to confirm the entry point of the wire as well as the entrance of the occlusion when necessary.

In addition, when using a parallel wiring technique, the wires occasionally enlarge the subintimal space in difficult CTO procedures. Once the subintimal space expands beyond the distal end of the CTO, the distal true lumen can be hardly seen in fluoroscopy. In these situations we often have to abandon the subsequent procedure when only the angiographical guidance is used. However, IVUS has a potential to make a breakthrough in these situations. If you deliver an IVUS catheter through the wire in the subintimal space, the IVUS image clearly shows important cross-sectional information: the IVUS catheter, a wire in the subintimal space, and a collapsed true channel. The next step is to introduce another wire into the true channel under IVUS guidance. IVUS visualizes the direction of

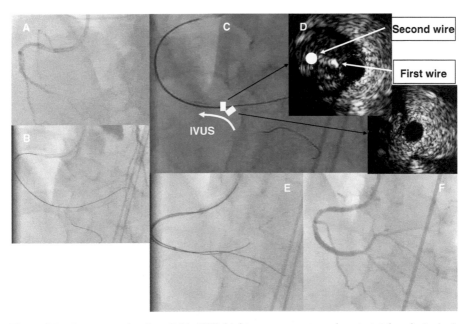

Figure 3.7 Case example of an RCA CTO (right coronary artery chronic total occlusion). A middle-aged female patient with angina. The first attempt at revascularization of the right coronary CTO (A) failed. In the second attempt, the first wire (intermediate) easily went out of the true channel (B). An intravasculor ultrasound (IVUS) image from the proximal small branch (C) clearly showed that the entry point of the first wire was too close to the branch (D), so that it easily advanced in the subintimal space. The correct position of the entry point for the second wire is in the center of the obstructed true channel, directly opposite to the branch origin. So the course of the next wire was intentionally changed from the CTO entrance towards the opposite direction to the branch angiographically. This wire easily got into the distal small branch (E). Final angiographic result after stenting (F). Such corrective action could be undertaken only by IVUS guidance.

the true channel and the entry point from the subintimal space into the true lumen so that we can attempt to reach it with a stiff wire. A typical case is shown in Figure 3.8.

On the other hand, some drawbacks and pitfalls in this procedure should be mentioned:

1. To deliver an IVUS catheter through the subintimal space, a balloon dilatation is sometimes required.
2. When a major perforation from the subintimal space is already observed, never move on to this technique.
3. A big guiding catheter is needed to be able to deliver an IVUS catheter and the support catheter/crossing wire system simultaneously.
4. To puncture the subintimal space, a sharp-cut stiff wire should be used, such as a tapered stiff wire (Confianza, Asahi Intec, Japan).
5. Multiple stenting is mandatory after successful puncturing to fully cover the extended subintimal space.

Finally, this procedure is not always successful. In our experience the success rate is around 60%. The encouraging message is that we can retrieve more than

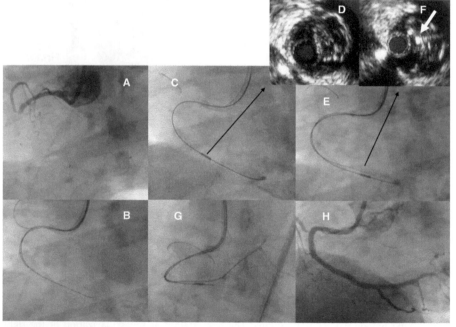

Figure 3.8 Case example of an RCA CTO (right coronary artery chronic total occlusion). An elderly male patient with angina and an old myocardial infarction. The RCA had a very long occlusion and was 3 years after occlusive instent restenosis (A). The parallel wiring technique using stiff wires could not provide successful wire crossing (B). An IVUS catheter was advanced through the wire in the false channel (C). The image clearly showed an expanded false lumen and a collapsed true channel (D). The next step was to penetrate the true lumen from the false channel by using a stiff wire. A Confianza wire made repeated attempts under IVUS guidance, and finally this procedure was successful (E, F). Following this, the wire was carefully advanced to the distal true channel (G). Final angiographic result after stenting is shown in panel H.

half of angiographical failure cases by using IVUS. Thus, this technique could be one of the last alternatives when standard wiring procedures fail.

CONCLUSIONS

Several specialized techniques can complement the classic single-wire manipulation in a CTO. The parallel wire technique takes advantage of the lessons learned during passage of the first wire into the subintimal space, and uses that wire as a continuous landmark. A more aggressive alternative is the seesaw technique, which includes alternating manipulations of two-wire systems within the subintimal space using each other as landmarks, but with a greater chance of compressing the true channel than the parallel wire method. Anchoring of the guide, using a balloon catheter, increases support. IVUS imaging can identify the CTO entry when no stump is visible, and can help to locate the true channel when inserted in the subintimal space.

4

Retrograde and bilateral techniques

Jean-François Surmely and Osamu Katoh

Suitable channel for the retrograde approach • Relevance of histopathology of CTOs
to the retrograde approach • Description of retrograde technique • Reaching the
distal end of the CTO with a retrograde wire • Controlled Antegrade and Retrograde
subintimal Tracking (CART) technique • Significance of septal collateral
dilatation • Indications and limitations of the retrograde approach • Conclusions

Percutaneous treatment of coronary total occlusions remains one of the major
challenges in interventional cardiology. Recent data have shown that successful
percutaneous recanalization of chronic total occlusions (CTOs) results in improved
survival, as well as enhanced left ventricular function, reduction in angina, and
improved exercise tolerance.[1-3] However, because of the perceived procedural
complexity of angioplasty in CTOs, it still represents the most common reason
for referral to bypass surgery, or for choosing medical treatment.[4,5] Over the past
few years, tremendous improvements in the PCI (percutaneous coronary intervention) equipment and materials, as well as the growth of new treatment strategies, have allowed us to tackle with success even complex CTO cases.

In this chapter on the retrograde approach for the percutaneous revascularization of CTOs, we first give an overview of some basic knowledge about coronary
collateral channels, as well as the relevant histopathological features of CTOs,
before focusing on the description of the three techniques using a retrograde
approach.

SUITABLE CHANNEL FOR THE RETROGRADE APPROACH

The retrograde approach requires a channel between the occluded coronary
artery and another patent coronary artery, which enables the distal CTO site to
be reached in a retrograde way. The intercoronary channel can be either an epicardial collateral, a septal collateral, or a bypass graft.

Anatomical classification of collaterals

In the human heart, the major epicardial coronary arteries and their branches
communicate with one another by means of anastomotic channels called collaterals.

If stenosis of an epicardial coronary artery produces a pressure gradient across such a channel, the collateral may become functional.

Our current knowledge on the anatomy and development of collaterals is based upon autopsy studies[6] or angiographic studies.[7-9] Using plastic casts of coronary arteries obtained in both normal and pathological human hearts, Baroldi showed that in normal coronaries there are innumerable collaterals with a diameter of 20–350 µm, and with a corkscrew aspect. The number of collaterals and their diameter (up to a maximum of 1 mm) are increased in significant coronary artery disease (CAD) (Figure 4.1). Baroldi proposed a classification based on the relationship between the donor and recipient artery as follows:

- Homocoronary collaterals that connect segments of the same artery.
- between branches of the same artery, or within the same branch.
- Intercoronary collaterals that connect branches of different arteries.[6]

The limited resolution of angiography does not allow visualization of very small collateral channels. In early studies, collaterals were seen angiographically only when a severe narrowing (>90%) or a total occlusion was present.[7,8] Based on this careful analysis, Levin described 26 different collateral pathways. Based on a recent angiographic assessment of collateral connection in patients with CTO using an angiographic system with a 0.2 mm resolution, two further classifications have been proposed. The anatomical course of the principal collateral is through septal connections (between septal perforators of anterior and posterior descending arteries) in 44%, atrial epicardial connections in 32%, distal interarterial connections in 18%, and bridging connections in 6%. According to the size of the collaterals, there was no visible continuous connection between donor and recipient artery in 14%, a continuous thread-like connection (<0.3 mm) in 51%, and a continuous small side branch-like size of the collateral throughout its course (>0.4 mm) in 35%.[9]

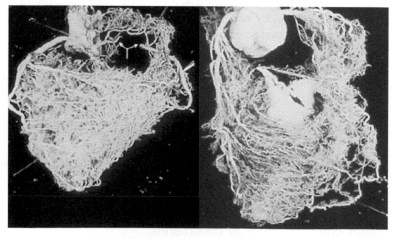

Figure 4.1   Coronary arteries plastic cast in a case of right coronary CTO. Left panel: numerous homo- and intercoronary collaterals are seen on the anterior wall. Right panel: image showing numerous continuous septal collaterals. (Courtesy of Dr Giorgio Baroldi.)

In order to be used as a retrograde channel for a percutaneous CTO intervention, the collateral should be visualized throughout its course, which is a common finding in CTOs (86%), as noted in the study by Werner et al.[9] This is nowadays probably even more frequently observed, with the improved resolution of the most recent angiographic systems available.

Histology of collaterals

Small collaterals with a diameter <0.5 mm are principally capillary-like, with no or rare smooth muscle. Bigger collaterals are principally arteriolar-like, with a thin muscular tunica media, a thin fibrous adventitial sheath, and an internal elastic membrane present only focally.[6]

Coronary collateral development

Augmentation of the collateral circulation is achieved by collateral recruitment or arteriogenesis. Collateral recruitment means that preexisting collateral vessels increase their lumen due to a change in vascular tone. Arteriogenesis indicates the development of capillary-like collaterals into arteriolar-like collaterals. Arteriogenesis occurs when a high-grade coronary stenosis is present. The mechanisms include endothelial proliferation, smooth muscle proliferation, and proteolytic activity to create the space for the expanding vessel and remodel the structures of the vessel itself.[10,11]

RELEVANCE OF HISTOPATHOLOGY OF CTOS TO THE RETROGRADE APPROACH

Chronic coronary total occlusions arise predominantly on a thrombotic occlusion. Thrombus organization and tissue aging then modify the tissue composition of CTOs over time. CTO tissue consists of intracellular and extracellular lipids, smooth muscle cells, loose or dense fibrous tissue (collagens), calcium, and neovascular channels. The concentration of collagen-rich fibrous tissue is particularly dense at the proximal CTO part and loose at its distal end.[12-14] A CTO lesion is therefore composed of a proximal and distal fibrous cap surrounding a softer core of organized thrombus and lipids (body of CTO). The proximal fibrous cap is thicker and harder than the distal fibrous cap (Figure 4.2). The distal fibrous cap is typically tapered. When looked at from the proximal side, the distal fibrous cap has therefore a convex shape. These features often make the penetration of the distal cap in an antegrade manner problematic (Figure 4.3). These two characteristics (thin, tapered) of the distal fibrous cap, have been of paramount importance for the development and successful application of the retrograde approach for percutaneous CTO recanalization.

DESCRIPTION OF RETROGRADE TECHNIQUE

Percutaneous CTO recanalization was first attempted in the 1980s. With increased operator experience and improved PCI material and technique, a success rate of between 50 and 70% could be achieved with the use of the standard techniques.

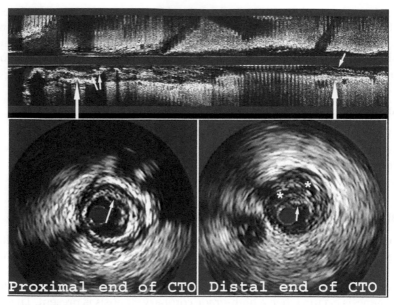

Figure 4.2 Longitudinal (upper panel) and cross-sectional intravascular ultrasound (IVUS) views illustrating the differences between the proximal and distal fibrous caps in a case of an old proximal LAD CTO (left anterior descending artery chronic total occlusion). IVUS recording was performed post dilatation with a 1.5 mm balloon. The corresponding locations of the proximal CTO end (left lower panel) and of the distal CTO end (right lower panel) on the longitudinal view are indicated with a thick white arrow. A dense fibrous cap surrounded by calcification is seen at the proximal occlusion end. The distal cap is very thin. False lumen due to failure of penetrating the distal cap can be seen (*). Fibrous caps are shown with thin white arrows.

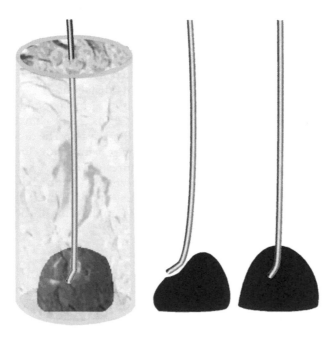

Figure 4.3 The shape of the distal fibrous cap is often dome-shaped (convex). When the wire tip reaches this dome-shaped distal fibrous cap, it often fails to penetrate and cross it into the distal true lumen, but instead slides along it into the subintimal space. It is important to review the position of the wire tip with the distal true lumen at different angles, because a subintimal location of the wire tip can be misleading in certain projections.

In order to improve this, still suboptimal, success rate, the retrograde approach was introduced. The first technique introduced that used a retrograde approach was the retrograde wire technique, then the kissing wire technique, and more recently the Controlled Antegrade and Retrograde subintimal Tracking technique (CART technique). The retrograde approach requires a channel between the occluded coronary artery and another patent coronary artery, which enables the distal CTO site to be reached retrogradely. This intercoronary channel can be either an epicardial collateral, a septal collateral, or a bypass graft. Meticulous review of the angiography, frame by frame, frequently allows a suitable collateral channel to be identified. In most cases, septal collaterals are considered to be the most suitable, as described later.

Retrograde wire technique

This recanalization technique uses a retrograde approach with a single wire, without simultaneous antegrade approach. The CTO is crossed only in a retrograde manner. The success rate of such a procedure is relatively low. Owing to the long access route of the retrograde wire via an intercoronary channel, its maneuverability is poor, and it is difficult to lead it through the CTO lesion. In addition, dissection occurring in the proximal vessel part can compromise an important side branch. Nowadays, this technique is largely abandoned, apart from the case of ostial CTOs, where it still has a role to play.

Kissing wire technique

This technique combines the simultaneous use of antegrade and retrograde approaches. The retrograde wire serves either as a marker of the distal CTO location or creates an intraluminal channel in the distal CTO portion. This facilitates the passage of a second intraluminal wire in an antegrade direction until they meet ('kiss') each other. This technique was often used for a retrograde approach before the CART and septal dilation technique had been established. Currently, this technique is only used if the CART technique cannot be performed due to failure of bringing an over-the-wire (OTW) balloon catheter through the intercoronary channel.

Controlled Antegrade and Retrograde subintimal Tracking technique (CART technique)

This technique combines the simultaneous use of antegrade and retrograde approaches. The basic concept of the CART technique is to create a subintimal dissection with limited extension, only at the site of the CTO. The procedure will be described in detail below.

REACHING THE DISTAL END OF THE CTO WITH A RETROGRADE WIRE

Technical steps

A guiding catheter is placed in the vessel with the occlusion, as well as in the other coronary artery from which the collateral channel arises. Following injection of a vasodilator, a soft wire, preferably hydrophilic, is advanced through the inter-coronary collateral with a microcatheter, in order to protect the channel from injury, maintain superb wire maneuverability, and perform a superselective injection.

After this wire and the microcatheter are placed in the collateral channel, a superselective injection is done to identify the channel course and anatomy. According to this precise angiographic map, the retrograde wire with a tiny

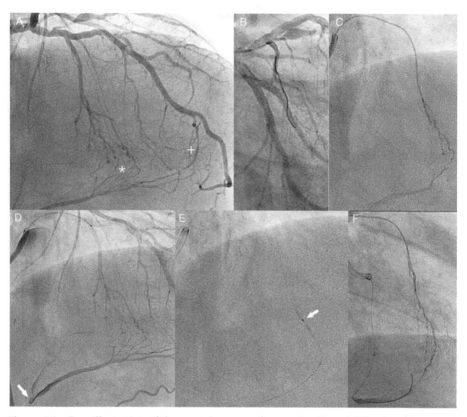

Figure 4.4 Case illustration of the procedure steps for septal collateral dilatation. The septal collateral course is difficult to identify on a non-selective injection of the contralateral patent coronary artery, owing to superposition with other collaterals. Two continuous collaterals can be seen. The targeted collateral originates from a septal perforator in the proximal left anterior descending artery (*); a second collateral (+) originates from the distal left anterior descending artery (panel A). A hydrophilic floppy wire is advanced in the proximal portion of the septal branch from which originates the most suitable collateral (panel B). A microcatheter is advanced until the tip of the wire, and the wire is pulled out. A superselective contrast injection of the septal collateral is then performed (panel C). The hydrophilic floppy wire is then advanced through the septal collateral with the microcatheter, in order to protect the channel from injury as well as to obtain a better wire maneuverability. A contralateral non-selective injection verifies the intraluminal location of the wire, which reached the distal end of the CTO (white arrow, panel D). The microcatheter is pulled out, and a small balloon (white arrow) is then advanced in the septal collateral, where sequential low-pressure dilatation is performed (panel E). A superselective contrast injection is recorded at the end of the procedure (panel F).

Surmely JF, Katoh O, Tsuchikane E, Nasu K, and Suzuki T. 2007. Coronary septal collaterals as an access for the retrograde approach in the percutaneous treatment of coronary chronic total occlusions. Catherization and Cardiovascular Interventions 2007; 69: 826 * 832.

curve at the tip is gently handled to pass through the channel. A polymer wire with a hydrophilic coating is the best for this procedure. Advancing the microcatheter step by step behind the wire is required for delicate wire handling. After the wire is passed through the channel, the microcatheter is exchanged for an OTW balloon catheter (Figure 4.4). The tip of the OTW balloon should be placed in the vessel segment where the CTO ends in order to visualize at best the distal anatomy of the CTO via a superselective injection, as well as to get a better wire maneuverability and support. In case of a septal collateral, dilation of the channel with a 1.25 mm balloon is usually required for the catheter to get through the channel, as described later.

Penetration of the distal fibrous cap from the distal true lumen into the CTO is attempted. If the wire is too soft for penetrating into the CTO or it is difficult to approach the end of the CTO due to poor wire maneuverability, inflation of the OTW balloon in the segment distal to the CTO (anchor) is helpful to overcome this difficulty. Exchange via the OTW balloon for stiffer wires can be done. The distal fibrous cap morphology is often soft and tapered when viewed from the distal lumen, which makes it easier to perforate it retrogradely than antegradely, so that stiffer wire is usually unnecessary. The wire handling follows the same recommendations as for the conventional single-wire antegrade technique.

Tips and tricks

1. A superselective contrast injection via a microcatheter or OTW balloon catheter is mandatory to confirm the channel course as well as its *continuous* character.
2. The chosen intercoronary channel should be located at least a few millimeters more distally than the distal CTO end. This allows having a coaxial position of the wire tip in relation to the distal CTO cap (Figure 4.5).

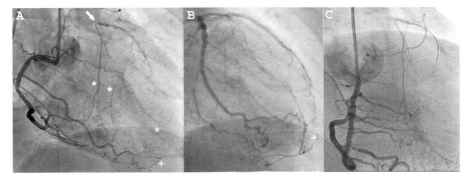

Figure 4.5 Right (panel A) and left (panel B) baseline coronary angiograms in an LAD CTO (left anterior descending artery chronic total occlusion) case. Several continuous collaterals can be seen (* = septal collaterals; + = epicardial collaterals). Epicardial collaterals have a long tortuous course with some acute bendings and focal narrowing. The first and biggest septal collateral reaches the LAD just at the CTO end (white arrow), which makes wire manipulation difficult. A more distal continuous septal collateral was chosen for the retrograde approach, which allows a coaxial wire position to be reached with the course of the CTO vessel (panel C).

Table 4.1	Recommended equipment for the retrograde approach
Guiding catheter	• Short guiding catheter (80–85 cm) • Brachial approach might be required in tall patients • 6–8 Fr
Wire	• Polymer wire with hydrophilic coating for the navigation through the tortuous intercoronary channel • Stiff wire is usually not required for getting retrogradely into the CTO
Microcatheter	• Superselective injection is necessary to look for suitable channel • Required for step-by-step wire navigation and protection of the intercoronary channel
Balloon	• Over-the-wire balloon with longer shaft of 150–155 cm (if normal guiding catheters are used) • Low-profile balloon • 1.25 mm size for septal dilatation • Size from 1.5–2.5 mm for CTO site dilatation

Pitfalls

1. Specific equipment is required because of the increased intra-arterial length that the wire and balloon catheter need to span (Table 4.1).
2. The parallel wire technique cannot be applied retrogradely.
3. Complications secondary to thrombosis (due to long stasis), or to the handling of the guiding catheter, guidewire, and balloon catheter may occur in the patent coronary artery from which the intercoronary collateral arises.

CONTROLLED ANTEGRADE AND RETROGRADE SUBINTIMAL TRACKING (CART) TECHNIQUE

Concept and clinical experience

This technique combines the simultaneous use of antegrade and retrograde approaches. The basic concept of the CART technique is to create a subintimal dissection with limited extension, only at the site of the CTO (Figure 4.6).

In the first 10 patients we treated with the CART technique, which included old and difficult CTOs (repeated treatment was attempted in 8 of the 10 patients), successful vessel recanalization was obtained in all cases. The intercoronary collateral used for the retrograde approach was a septal branch in four cases and a collateral between the circumflex artery and the posterolateral branch of the distal right coronary artery in five cases. In one case, the retrograde approach was performed through a bypass graft (gastroepiploic artery) to the posterior descending artery of the right coronary. No complications such as perforation or occlusion occurred in the collateral channel. In all cases, the subintimal dissection was limited in the CTO region.

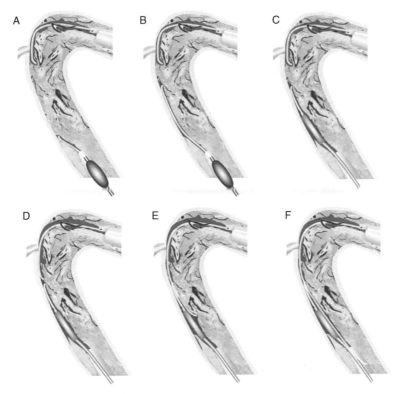

Figure 4.6 Schema of the different steps for the Controlled Antegrade and Retrograde subintimal Tracking (CART) technique. (A) First, a wire is advanced antegradely from the proximal true lumen into the CTO, then into the subintimal space at the CTO site. Then, a retrograde wire with an over-the-wire (OTW) balloon is advanced retrogradely from the distal true lumen into the CTO. (B) The retrograde wire is further advanced into the subintimal space at the CTO site. (C) Balloon dilatation of the subintimal space and also on the course from this subintimal space to the distal end of the CTO. The deflated balloon is left in place. (D and E) The antegrade wire is further advanced in the subintimal space until it connects with the retrograde wire. (F) The antegrade wire is advanced through the channel made by the retrograde wire into the distal true lumen.

Surmely JF, Tsuchikane E, Katoh O, Nishida Y, Nakayama M, Nakamura S, Oida A, Hattori E, and Suzuki T. 2006. New concept for CTO recanalization using controlled antegrade and retrograde subintimal tracking: the CART technique. Journal of Invasive Cardiology 2006; 18:334–338. Reprinted with permission from the Journal of Invasive Cardiology. 2006; 18:334–338. Copyright HMP Communications.

Technical steps

First, a wire is advanced antegradely from the proximal true lumen into the CTO, then into the subintimal space at the CTO site. Experienced operators can recognize the wire entering into the subintimal space by a decreased resistance of the wire tip or wire movement.

Secondly, another wire is advanced through the intercoronary collateral with a microcatheter, in order to protect the channel from injury as well as to obtain better wire maneuverability. This wire is placed at the distal end of the CTO, and then penetrates retrogradely from the distal true lumen into the CTO, then into the subintimal space at the CTO site.

After advancing a small balloon (1.5–2.5 mm) over the retrograde wire into the subintima, the balloon should be inflated in the subintima and also on the course from this subintimal space to the distal end of the CTO. In order to keep this subintimal space open, the deflated balloon should be left in place. As a consequence, the two dissections created by the antegrade wire and the retrograde balloon lie in the subintima at the CTO site (Figure 4.7), which allows us to connect

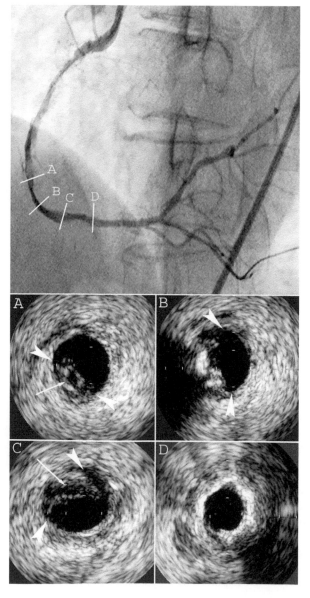

Figure 4.7 Intravascular ultrasound images obtained after recanalization and balloon dilatation of a long and old right coronary artery CTO in which the CART technique was performed. Sequential images illustrating the passage from the subintimal space (A, B, and C) to the distal true lumen (D). The arrowheads show the extension of the large subintimal dissection. The arrows show the CTO tissue located next to the dissection plane.
Surmely JF, Tsuchikane E, Katoh O, Nishida Y, Nakayama M, Nakamura S, Oida A, Hattori E, and Suzuki T. 2006. New concept for CTO recanalization using controlled antegrade and retrograde subintimal tracking: the CART technique. Journal of Invasive Cardiology 2006; 18:334–338. Reprinted with permission from the Journal of Invasive Cardiology. 2006; 18:334–338. Copyright HMP Communications.

both of them easily. Thereafter, the antegrade wire is advanced further along the deflated retrograde balloon, which lies from the subintimal space to the distal true lumen. This technique allows a limited subintimal tracking situated only in the portion of the CTO lesion, and avoids the difficulty of reentering the distal true lumen. After successful recanalization, dilatation and stent implantation are performed. The different steps of the procedure are illustrated in Figure 4.6, and case examples are given in Figures 4.8 and 4.9.

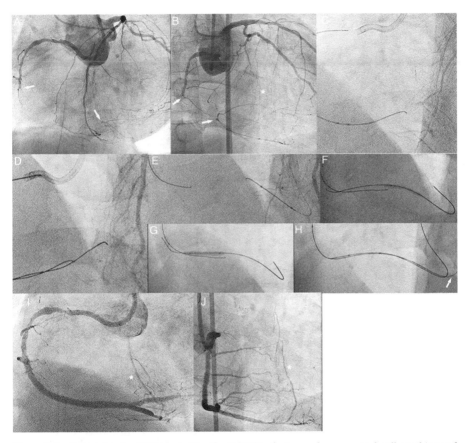

Figure 4.8 Example of a CTO treated by the CART technique where a septal collateral is used as an intercoronary channel. Baseline findings obtained by bilateral injection show a long right coronary CTO. White arrows show the proximal and distal occlusion end (panel A, left anterior oblique [LAO] view; panel B, right anterior oblique [RAO] view; * indicates the septal collateral used later for the retrograde approach). An antegrade approach was first attempted with a single wire (C), then with the parallel wire technique (D), but failed to puncture the distal CTO cap. A retrograde wire was advanced through a septal collateral channel up to the distal CTO end (E). Penetration of the CTO end was achieved, and balloon dilatations at the bifurcation of the distal right coronary artery, the posterior descending artery, as well as in the distal right coronary segment were performed over the retrograde wire (F and G). Thereafter, the antegrade wire (white arrow) could be placed easily in the posterior descending artery (H). The rest of the procedure was then performed in an antegrade manner with balloon dilatation of the CTO site followed by stent implantation. The final result is shown in panels I and J. The dilated septal collateral used for the retrograde approach is clearly seen (*) in those final views.

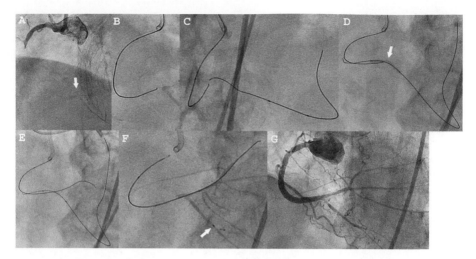

Figure 4.9 Example of a right coronary CTO treated by the CART technique where a septal collateral is used as an intercoronary channel. Baseline finding obtained by bilateral injection (A). The distal end of the CTO (white arrow) can be seen via the contralateral injection. An antegrade approach was first attempted, but the antegrade wire could not puncture the distal CTO cap (B). A retrograde wire was advanced through a septal collateral channel up to the distal CTO end (C). Penetration of the CTO end was achieved, and balloon dilatation (white arrow) at the bifurcation of the distal right coronary artery was performed over the retrograde wire (D). Thereafter, the antegrade wire could be placed easily in the posterolateral branch of the right coronary artery (E). The retrograde wire was pulled out and a superselective injection via the over-the-wire (OTW) balloon (white arrow) was done to confirm the intraluminal position of the antegrade wire (F). Balloon dilatation of the CTO site followed by stent implantation was then performed with a good final result (G).
Surmely JF, Katoh O, Tsuchikane E, Nasu K, and Suzuki T. 2007. Coronary septal collaterals as an access for the retrograde approach in the percutaneous treatment of coronary chronic total occlusions. Catheterization and Cardiovascular Interventions 2007; 69: 826 * 832.

Tips and tricks

1. To facilitate antegrade wire passage into the subintimal space, the antegrade wire should be manipulated to aim directly at the balloon left in the subintimal space. The tip of the wire touching the balloon tends to automatically slip into the subintimal space along the balloon track.
2. An antegrade flow should be confirmed after balloon dilatation of the entire CTO length over the antegrade wire. An antegrade flow should be obtained before pulling out the retrograde wire.

SIGNIFICANCE OF SEPTAL COLLATERAL DILATATION

As mentioned previously, the retrograde approach requires an intercoronary channel, which can be either an epicardial collateral, a septal collateral, or a bypass graft. The big diameter of a bypass graft makes the wire manipulation relatively easy. However, the risk of damaging the graft, particularly for a venous graft, can have disastrous consequences. The risk of potentially jeopardizing a functioning graft must be carefully weighed against the benefit of a successful CTO recanalization, which cannot be achieved in an antegrade approach.

Epicardial collaterals of moderate size are present in about 50% of CTOs:[9] they are often corkscrew-like and often have a focal diameter narrowing (stricture/stenosis) at bending sites. This can make advancement of a balloon catheter very difficult if not impossible. In addition, bleeding secondary to perforation of an epicardial collateral can be difficult to stop, and can result in a large pericardial effusion that needs emergency surgical intervention.

Collaterals with an intramuscular course are therefore preferred. Intraseptal collaterals run either inside the septal myocardium or under the endocardium. Perforation of a septal collateral, which is surrounded by myocardium, will in most cases stop bleeding after a long balloon inflation or even spontaneously. When the septal collateral is running subendocardially, perforation can create a communication with the left or the right ventricle (Figure 4.10). Such a communication will result in a physiologically non-significant shunt and will probably disappear due to the differences of pressure between the ventricles and the septal collateral.

A collateral with continuous small side branch-like size throughout its course is found in only one-fourth of the cases. However, a continuous connection is found in more than 80% of the cases. The use of such small collaterals necessitates a predilatation with a small balloon (1.25 mm), to allow its passage up to the distal CTO site. In a small series of 38 patients in whom retrograde CTO recanalization was recently attempted, septal collaterals were most frequently used as a retrograde access route (84%; 32/38). A guidewire successfully passed through the septal collateral channel in 88% (28/32) of cases and the channel was successfully dilated with a small balloon (1.25 or 1.5 mm balloon) in 26 of the 32 cases (81%). Channel rupture occurred in two cases (Figures 4.10 and 4.11). No specific treatment was needed, as they resulted in a small shunt between the septal collateral and ventricles without intraseptum hemorrhage. These data suggest that a septal channel can be safely used as an access route for the retrograde approach in most of the CTOs located in the right coronary or left anterior descending artery (personal data).

INDICATIONS AND LIMITATIONS OF THE RETROGRADE APPROACH

With the use of the standard techniques, a success rate of 50–70% can be achieved. The most common reason for CTO attempt failure is the inability to successfully pass a guidewire across the lesion into the true lumen of the distal vessel.[15] After guidewire penetration of the proximal CTO fibrous cap, the guidewire often enters the subintima, creating a subintimal lumen. Repeated wire manipulations in order to redirect the guidewire into the CTO body can result in extensive subintimal dissection, with accompanying extramural hematoma. Such dissections extend circumferentially and longitudinally and can compress the distal true lumen, which makes (at times) distal true lumen re-entry difficult. Another common reason for the unsuccessful recanalization is the difficulty of perforating the CTO distal fibrous cap, the guidewire sliding consequently into the subintimal space.

An antegrade approach should always be tried first with the parallel wire technique. If a favorable collateral anatomy is present, a retrograde approach can then be attempted and the shape and characteristics of the distal fibrous cap significantly increases the chances of successful recanalization. The septal collateral

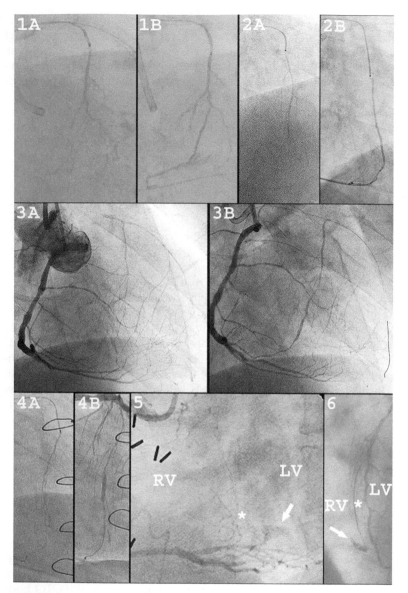

Figure 4.10 Examples of pre- and postseptal collateral dilatation. Case 1: on the predilatation superselective injection (1A), the collateral continuity is just visible. The postdilatation result is shown on panel 1B. Case 2: the collateral continuity cannot be clearly visualized (2A); postdilatation result (2B). Case 3: on the predilatation non-selective injection, several continuous collaterals are clearly seen (3A). Postdilatation result (3B). Septal collateral complications are shown on the following three cases. Case 4: example of an aneurysm postseptal dilatation (4A, predilatation image; 4B, postdilatation image). Case 5: septal collateral perforation (white arrow) communicating with the left ventricle (LV). The position of the interventricular septum is indicated by the presence of septal collaterals (*). Case 6: septal collateral perforation (white arrow) communicating with the right ventricle (RV).

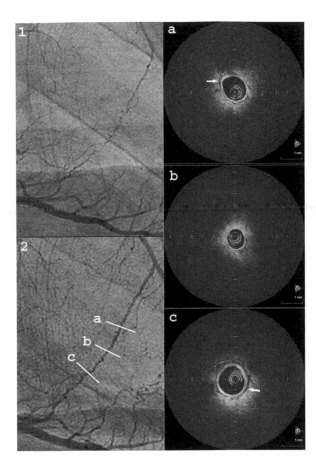

Figure 4.11 Predilatation (panel 1) and postdilatation (panel 2) images of septal collateral. Postseptal dilatation, optical coherence tomography images were recorded (panels a, b, and c) and their locations are shown on panel 2. Image b is located at the junction site between the septal perforator artery originating from the left anterior descending artery and the posterior descending branch from the right coronary artery. At this site, the collateral is capillary-like without the presence of smooth muscle cells. Images a and c are situated proximally and distally from the junction site and have an arteriolar-like morphology. Postdilatation dissection (white arrow) can be seen behind the muscular layer.
Surmely JF, Katoh O, Tsuchikane E, Nasu K, and Suzuki T. 2007. Coronary spetal collaterals as an access for the retrograde approach in the percutaneous treatment of coronary chronic total occlusions. Catheterization and Cardiovascular Interventions 2007; 69: 826 * 832.

dilation technique has greatly expanded the indication of the retrograde approach and a high success rate for recanalization is achieved with the CART technique.

Our current experience shows that in 80% of CTOs in the right coronary or left anterior descending artery, the retrograde approach can be applied if necessary and the CART technique is successful in more than 90% of those cases. The percutaneous dilatation of the septal collateral and the CART technique provide new horizons in the percutaneous approach of CTOs, ensuring high procedural success. Potential complications include ischemia during the procedure (spasm or thrombosis in the proximal target vessel or the collateral-providing vessel), damaging the intercoronary channel such as perforation or abrupt closure, as well as complications secondary to the handling of the guiding catheter, guidewire, and balloon catheter in the patent coronary artery from which arises the intercoronary collateral.

CONCLUSIONS

Data obtained over the past decade have provided a growing body of evidence demonstrating that a successful percutaneous recanalization of a coronary chronic total occlusion translates into a clinical benefit. However, because of the perceived procedural complexity of angioplasty in CTOs, the condition still represents the most common reason for referral to bypass surgery, or for choosing medical treatment.

The proven clinical benefit, as well as the improved long-term patency with drug-eluting stents,[16-19] has resulted in a growing interest among interventional cardiologists for treating CTOs. Over the past few years, tremendous improvements in the PCI equipment, and the development of innovative strategies, have allowed very high success rates, even in complex CTO cases. Every strategy has its advantages as well as its disadvantages.

To avoid complications and therefore putting the patient at risk, it is extremely important to understand the principles of each strategy and to be able to handle the necessary equipment appropriately, and, before everything, to be aware of the limitations and possible complications of each technique. It is also important to know how long we should try a technique before switching to more complex techniques. In this chapter we outlined the indications and procedural steps of the retrograde approach. Personal experience has led to the introduction of the CART technique and of the percutaneous septal collateral dilatation. Those techniques have been both feasible and safe, and most importantly, they increase significantly the success rate in percutaneous CTOs recanalization.

REFERENCES

1. Melchior JP, Doriot PA, Chatelain P, et al. Improvement of left ventricular contraction and relaxation synchronism after recanalization of chronic total coronary occlusion by angioplasty. J Am Coll Cardiol 1987; 9(4):763–8.
2. Olivari Z, Rubartelli P, Piscione F, et al. Immediate results and one-year clinical outcome after percutaneous coronary interventions in chronic total occlusions: data from a multicenter, prospective, observational study (TOAST-GISE). J Am Coll Cardiol 2003; 41(10):1672–8.
3. Suero JA, Marso SP, Jones PG, et al. Procedural outcomes and long-term survival among patients undergoing percutaneous coronary intervention of a chronic total occlusion in native coronary arteries: a 20-year experience. J Am Coll Cardiol 2001; 38(2):409–14.
4. Bourassa MG, Roubin GS, Detre KM, et al. Bypass Angioplasty Revascularization Investigation: patient screening, selection, and recruitment. Am J Cardiol 1995; 75(9):3C–8C.
5. King SB 3rd, Lembo NJ, Weintraub WS, et al. A randomized trial comparing coronary angioplasty with coronary bypass surgery. Emory Angioplasty versus Surgery Trial (EAST). N Engl J Med 1994; 331(16):1044–50.
6. Baroldi G. Functional morphology of the anastomotic circulation in human cardiac pathology. Methods Achiev Exp Pathol 1971; 5:438–73.
7. Gensini GG, Bruto da Costa BC. The coronary collateral circulation in living man. Am J Cardiol 1969; 24(3):393–400.
8. Levin DC. Pathways and functional significance of the coronary collateral circulation. Circulation 1974; 50(4):831–7.
9. Werner GS, Ferrari M, Heinke S, et al. Angiographic assessment of collateral connections in comparison with invasively determined collateral function in chronic coronary occlusions. Circulation 2003; 107(15):1972–7.
10. Fujita M, Tambara K. Recent insights into human coronary collateral development. Heart 2004; 90(3):246–50.
11. Schaper W, Ito WD. Molecular mechanisms of coronary collateral vessel growth. Circ Res 1996; 79(5):911–19.
12. Katsuragawa M, Fujiwara H, Miyamae M, Sasayama S. Histologic studies in percutaneous transluminal coronary angioplasty for chronic total occlusion: comparison of tapering and

abrupt types of occlusion and short and long occluded segments. J Am Coll Cardiol 1993; 21(3):604–11.

13. Srivatsa S, Holmes D Jr. The histopathology of angiographic chronic total coronary artery occlusions and changes in neovascular pattern and intimal plaque composition associated with progressive occlusion duration. J Invasive Cardiol 1997; 9(4):294–301.

14. Srivatsa SS, Edwards WD, Boos CM, et al. Histologic correlates of angiographic chronic total coronary artery occlusions: influence of occlusion duration on neovascular channel patterns and intimal plaque composition. J Am Coll Cardiol 1997; 29(5):955–63.

15. Kinoshita I, Katoh O, Nariyama J, et al. Coronary angioplasty of chronic total occlusions with bridging collateral vessels: immediate and follow-up outcome from a large single-center experience. J Am Coll Cardiol 1995; 26(2):409–15.

16. Ge L, Iakovou I, Cosgrave J, et al. Immediate and mid-term outcomes of sirolimus-eluting stent implantation for chronic total occlusions. Eur Heart J 2005; 26(11):1056–62.

17. Hoye A, Tanabe K, Lemos PA, et al. Significant reduction in restenosis after the use of sirolimus-eluting stents in the treatment of chronic total occlusions. J Am Coll Cardiol 2004; 43(11):1954–8.

18. Nakamura S, Muthusamy TS, Bae JH, et al. Impact of sirolimus-eluting stent on the outcome of patients with chronic total occlusions. Am J Cardiol 2005; 95(2):161–6.

19. Werner GS, Schwarz G, Prochnau D, et al. Paclitaxel-eluting stents for the treatment of chronic total coronary occlusions: a strategy of extensive lesion coverage with drug-eluting stents. Catheter Cardiovasc Interv 2006; 67(1):1–9.

5

Subintimal tracking and reentry: the STAR technique

Antonio Colombo and Goran Stankovic

The Subintimal Tracking and Reentry (STAR) technique • The two most commonly asked questions and concerns • Some tips and tricks

The most important task when reopening a total occlusion is to gain guidewire access into the lumen immediately distal to the occluded segment. If by any chance the guidewire creates a subintimal passage in the occluded segment, such a passage has to be as short as possible. If the true lumen reentry is not achieved until the subintimal passage reaches a site remote from the occlusion site, angioplasty or stenting may compromise flow in the side branches originating from the subintimal track.[1] The risk to extend distally any possible subintimal track demands early usage of techniques such as the parallel wire technique with the intent of gaining access into the true lumen.[2] Devices that have been developed to facilitate true lumen reentry offer the potential to overcome this limitation, increasing the immediate success in treating chronic total occlusions (CTOs).[3-5]

When all technical skills and devices available (mostly guidewires) have been exhausted, the operator will need to resort to alternative approaches. The idea to recanalize a difficult occlusion by creating a subintimal dissection which will reenter the true lumen of the vessel in a distal segment of the artery is the basic principle of a very much utilized technique in peripheral angioplasty of total occlusions.[6-13] The technique of subintimal angioplasty was used first in 1987, by Amman Bolia, when a subintimal channel was accidentally created while successfully treating a 15 cm popliteal occlusion. Bolia recognized the potential of this technique when the vessel remained patent in follow-up for over 9 years and the procedure was first described in 1989.[7] Since the Leicester Group's initial report, the experience with subintimal angioplasty has expanded to include more than a thousand patients and additional anatomical segments, including tibial and iliac vessels.[10]

The rationale for this approach comes from the fact that in the case of an occluded lumen the blood supply to the vessel wall decreases, creating a zone of less vital vessel wall at the level of the media, which is more vulnerable to dissection. This is not new and vascular surgeons always use this natural dissection plane when performing an endarterectomy. With the percutaneous subintimal recanalization technique, however, the atheroma remains in situ and a new channel is created around this core. It is postulated that subintimal angioplasty may be superior to conventional angioplasty.[11] The subintimal channel is theoretically free of endothelium and atheroma, while with routine angioplasty the injured endothelium and atheroma can serve as a nidus for platelet aggregation and thrombus formation in the short term and neointimal hyperplasia in the long term.[11]

THE SUBINTIMAL TRACKING AND REENTRY (STAR) TECHNIQUE[14]

When performing the STAR technique to recanalize a coronary artery, we start with a 1.5 mm over-the-wire balloon and first create a subintimal dissection. Sometimes the subintimal dissection is already present from a prior attempt. The dissection is usually created with a stiff wire such as Intermediate or Miraclebros 3g or 6g or Conquest/Confianza (Asahi Intec, Seto, Japan). It is important to use the stiff wire only to create the initial track of the dissection. Attempts to advance the stiff wire distally may increase the risk of perforation. As soon as a subintimal track has been visibly created, the balloon is advanced in such a track and the wire is changed with a hydrophilic wire such as Whisper or Pilot 50 (Guidant, Abbott). The hydrophilic wire is shaped with a pronounced J tip in order to be completely atraumatic when advanced into the dissection plane. The loop turns around the occluded lumen in a spiral fashion, guided by the softest areas in the subintimal space. The J-shaped configuration will allow staying in the dissection plane, minimizing the risks of perforation. In the subintimal plane, the guidewire assumes a characteristic 'wide loop' configuration, the diameter of which will appear similar to or larger than the luminal diameter of the artery. It is this loop which gains reentry into the true lumen distal to the occlusion. Reentry happens because the intima of the non-diseased segment is thinner. In this way we have created a device similar to the surgeon's ring stripper, and, like the surgeon, we proceed down through the natural dissection plane. Figure 5.1a–c presents a successful recanalization of the right coronary artery utilizing the STAR technique.

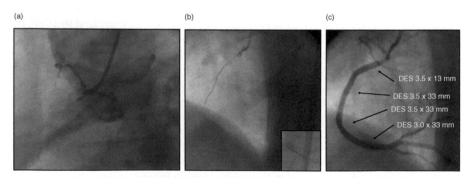

Figure 5.1   (a) Baseline angiogram shows occlusion of mid right coronary artery. (b) Dissection following recanalization. (c) Final result after stenting; DES, drug-eluting stent.

THE TWO MOST COMMONLY ASKED QUESTIONS AND CONCERNS

How do we prevent perforations?

It is possible to treat hard and calcified occlusions with subintimal angioplasty. However, to cross a hard occlusion, a degree of force is necessary and, in some cases, this leads to perforation. The risk of perforations in our experience has been small. As a matter of fact we have never had to perform pericardial drainage due to tamponade. If the operator maintains the loop while advancing the wire and keeps the loop small (short radius, Figure 5.2) by using a soft hydrophilic wire, especially when in a distal location, the risk of perforation remains very low. If in doubt, it is important to check with a retrograde injection that the wire direction is going in the appropriate anatomical site. In order to keep the loop relatively small and appropriate for the vessel size, we may use a stiff hydrophilic wire such as the Pilot 150 or 200 (Guidant, Abbott) proximally and use almost only the softer Whisper (Guidant, Abbott) when progressing more distally. As a rule of thumb, the diameter of the loop should be similar to the expected diameter of the media–media of the artery being treated.

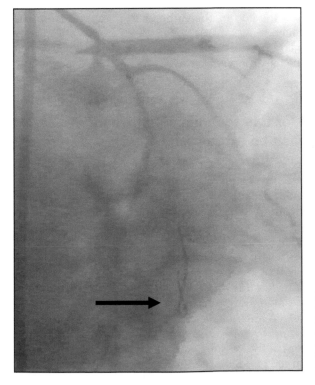

Figure 5.2 It is very important to maintain a closed and narrow loop, especially when advancing into small vessels. Arrow points to the classic loop of the wire in order to proceed in the subintimal spare.

How do we reenter into the true lumen when distally?

Reentering into the true lumen is almost an automatic phenomenon. Reentering occurs spontaneously when the wire is in a distal location. This happens presumably because the intima of the non-diseased segment is thinner. It seems that with advancement of the wire distally, a lower resistance is obtained toward the true lumen than towards the adventitia. When advancing the wire distally, the operator has to be careful about very distal perforations. We try not to advance the wire too distally unless we are sure we are following the true subintimal space. A good visualization from contralateral collaterals is important for this maneuver. As soon as the wire has reached a satisfactory intraluminal distal location, we advance the over-the-wire (OTW) balloon and we remove the hydrophilic wire and exchange it for a Balance Universal wire (Guidant, Abbott) in order to minimize the risk for any distal perforation.

The Pioneer catheter (Medtronic, Inc., Minneapolis, MN) or the Outback catheter (LuMend, Redwood City, CA, acquired by Cordis Corporation, Miami Lakes, FL), has been developed to facilitate true lumen reentry, allowing passage of a needle and guidewire across the intima distal to the occlusion.[5] The Pioneer catheter has intravascular ultrasound (IVUS) integrated into the device, which allows a real-time imaging at the time of needle deployment. In addition to showing the intima and true lumen, the color flow capability of IVUS imaging adds an additional confirmation of the patency of the vessel at the point of needle deployment.[3,15] The Outback catheter is a 5 Fr multipurpose-type angled guide catheter with an integral hypotube ending in a curved nitinol needle that can be advanced or retracted from the end of the catheter to penetrate from the dissection plane to the true lumen.[4]

These devices are useful in large vessels and are not particularly of help when employing the STAR technique in coronary arteries.

SOME TIPS AND TRICKS

Which vessel is suited for this technique and when should the STAR approach be attempted?

In order for the technique to be successful, the distal portion of the artery should be reasonably healthy. The presence of a disease-free distal segment allows reentry to be achieved and, more importantly, once an occlusion has been recanalized, the distal segment of the artery will have sufficient branches to allow an adequate distal runoff. Very diseased and poor distal segment beyond an occlusion is a relative contraindication for the STAR technique.

The most appropriate vessel where the STAR approach is utilized is the right coronary artery. The fact that the right coronary artery has few important branches proximal to the crux makes this procedure suitable. We performed the STAR with good immediate and follow-up results also on obtuse marginal branches (Figures 5.3a–d). The left anterior descending artery is most probably the least-suited vessel for this approach because most of the major branches are located in the proximal segment of the vessel. On some occasions we performed the STAR with good results in the mid left anterior descending artery provided patency and good flow is obtained towards at least two diagonal branches.

The STAR technique 53

(a)

(b)

(c)

DES 3.0 x 18 mm

DES 3.0 x 33 mm

DES 2.5 x 33 mm

(d)

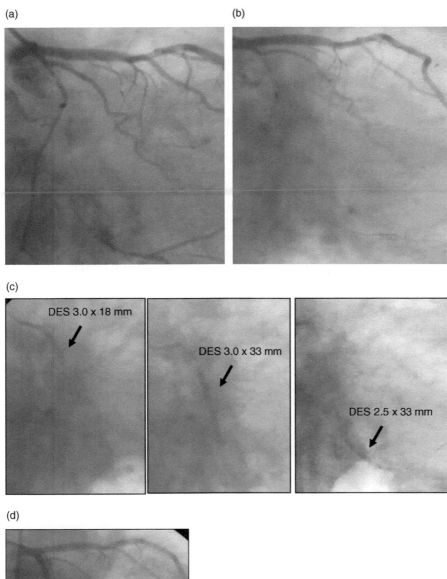

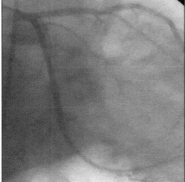

Figure 5.3 (a) Total occlusion of an obtuse marginal branch. (b) Reopening with subintimal dissection. (c) Placement of multiple stents; DES, drug-eluting stent. Arrows point to the origin of side branches (d) Final result.

In general, we rarely perform the STAR technique as the first-line procedure. Most of the time this approach is utilized when a prior attempt with a standard technique has failed or during a procedure in which a standard technique has created a large dissection. The operator may decide to convert the procedure into a STAR if the vessel and the clinical scenario are appropriate for this alternative solution.

What to do if the wire gains access into a minor branch?

If the wire gains access into a distal minor branch, we prefer to leave the wire there. We usually change the hydrophilic wire with a Balance Universal and then try to gain the distal lumen of the major vessel with a second wire. It is not rare that we use two or three wires and leave all of them in distal branches. What is important to keep in mind is that the long-time patency rate of the vessel reopened with the STAR technique depends on the number of vessels available for distal runoff. For this reason, we do not want to lose any opportunity to maintain access to any branch that could sustain good distal runoff. Most of the times we try to use an 8 Fr guiding catheter, which allows a more friendly operation with multiple wires in place.

What is the best way to gain access into side branches such as posterolateral branches, inferior descending artery, and branches of diagonals?

As shown in Figure 5.4, the origin of a side branch is frequently seen by the presence of a small nub or a dissection pointing into that direction. In other circumstances the origin of a side branch is only visible from collaterals visualized from the contralateral injection. Whatever opportunity we have available to visualize the origin of the side branch we use an OTW balloon with an intermediate wire or moderate stiff wire (Intermediate, or Miraclebros 3g; in rare situations Conquest/Confianza, Asahi Intec, Seto, Japan) to extend the dissection into the

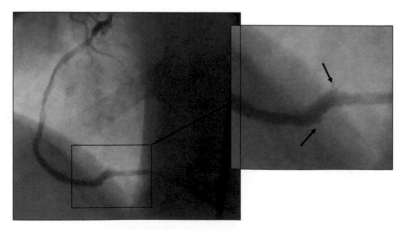

Figure 5.4   The origin of a side branch is seen by the presence of small nubs (arrows).

side branch (Figure 5.5). When the dissection has been extended a few millimeters to allow advancement of the balloon, we advance the balloon into the dissection created in the side branch and exchange the stiff wire for a Whisper wire with a tight J configuration. The Whisper wire is utilized to extend the dissection into the branch and, ultimately to obtain access to the distal lumen. Figure 5.6 shows the final result following stent implantation only proximally to the crux of the right coronary artery.

What can we do when reentry is not spontaneous?

Pull the wire back and try to find a new dissection plane.

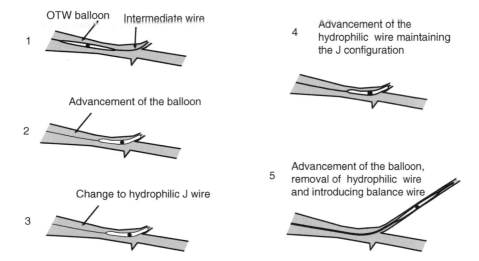

Figure 5.5 Recommended steps to gain access into the side branches: STAR performed inside the branches. OTW balloon, over-the-wire balloon.

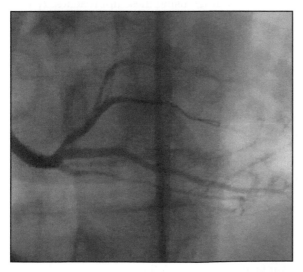

Figure 5.6 Final result following stent placement from the ostium to the crux; no stent was placed in the distal branches.

What size balloons do we use to perform dilatations prior to stenting?

We use balloons appropriately sized to the anatomical diameter of the vessel we are dilating and we inflate the balloon until we obtain full expansion. On rare occasions we need pressures over 10 atm to obtain full balloon expansion. In order to reduce any risk of vessel rupture (so far we have seen only contained ruptures and one case of pseudoaneurysm) we do not advise using a pressure over 12 atm in case the balloon does not fully expand.

When the time comes for stenting, how do we proceed?

First of all before proceeding to implant stents it is important to make sure that we have a sufficient good distal runoff. At least two branches runoff is important.

We usually stent from the proximal dissection plane, which coincides with the site of the original occlusion, until the first major bifurcation. Unless really necessary, we try to avoid bifurcational stenting. We are not afraid to leave distal dissections in the side branches as long as there is a good distal runoff.

When do we stent a bifurcation?

As stated above, we try to limit stenting to a segment proximal to a major bifurcation. For the right coronary artery we try not to stent distally to the crux. Despite this suggestion, there are conditions where, owing to the large size of the distal vessels and the presence of an unfavorable dissection involving a bifurcation, one or two stents are needed. We use one stent if we can determine that the dissection extends mainly towards one branch and the side branch is relatively free of dissections or, despite the presence of a dissection, has an optimal flow. When we need to implant two stents, we prefer to use a relatively simple technique. The complexity to re-cross into a side branch when performing a crush or culotte techniques can be such as to discourage using these approaches. A T or modified T is most probably the best way to reconstruct a distal bifurcation when needed with the lowest complexity to re-cross and to perform a final kissing inflation.

What type of stent should we utilize?

Drug-eluting stents are the most appropriate stents to be implanted.[14] The only limitation is the fact that, frequently, two or three stents or more are needed and this situation may pose financial problems.[16] We have occasionally utilized bare metal stents in the most proximal part of the vessel, where the reference diameter is large, and drug-eluting stents in the most distal part, where the reference vessel size is ≤3 mm. Overall, we are relatively pleased with this intermediate solution, even if our experience with this combined approach is limited, and whenever possible we try to use drug-eluting stents exclusively. Regarding the specific type of drug-eluting stent to be implanted, we have been using either Cypher (Cordis, a J&J Company, Miami Lakes, FL) or Taxus (Boston Scientific, Natick, MA) without any particular advantage of one vs the other.

For how long is double antiplatelet therapy continued?

We suggest a minimum of 1 year of double antiplatelet therapy. So far, no specific study has been performed to investigate the appropriate duration of double antiplatelet therapy. The fact that long and multiple stents have been implanted may suggest extending the duration of double antiplatelet therapy.

Should we perform angiographic follow-up and when?

We routinely suggest angiographic follow-up at 5–6 months from the procedure. If the distal runoff had at least two vessels, the vessel will maintain patency most of the times. In about 50% of cases, there is focal restenosis (Figures 5.7 and 5.8) that is treated by implantation of a short drug-eluting stent.

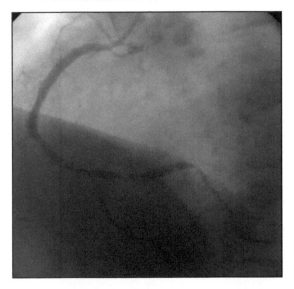

Figure 5.7   Multiple focal restenosis inside drug-eluting stents in the right coronary artery.

(a)   (b)

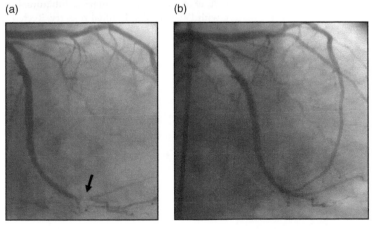

Figure 5.8   (a) Restenosis distal to multiple DES stents placed on an obtuse marginal branch. Arrow points to the site of distal restenosis (b) Final result following placement of an additional distal stent.

REFERENCES

1. Lipsitz EC, Ohki T, Veith FJ, et al. Fate of collateral vessels following subintimal angio-plasty. J Endovasc Ther 2004; 11:269–73.
2. Ochiai M, Ashida K, Araki H, et al. The latest wire technique for chronic total occlusion. Ital Heart J 2005; 6:489–93.
3. Casserly IP, Sachar R, Bajzer C, Yadav JS. Utility of IVUS-guided transaccess catheter in the treatment of long chronic total occlusion of the superficial femoral artery. Catheter Cardiovasc Interv 2004; 62:237–43.
4. Hausegger KA, Georgieva B, Portugaller H, Tauss J, Stark G. The outback catheter: a new device for true lumen re-entry after dissection during recanalization of arterial occlusions. Cardiovasc Intervent Radiol 2004; 27:26–30.
5. Jacobs DL, Motaganahalli RL, Cox DE, Wittgen CM, Peterson GJ. True lumen re-entry devices facilitate subintimal angioplasty and stenting of total chronic occlusions: initial report. J Vasc Surg 2006; 43:1291–6.
6. Bolia A, Sayers RD, Thompson MM, Bell PR. Subintimal and intraluminal recanalisation of occluded crural arteries by percutaneous balloon angioplasty. Eur J Vasc Surg 1994; 8:214–19.
7. Bolia A, Brennan J, Bell PR. Recanalisation of femoro-popliteal occlusions: improving success rate by subintimal recanalisation. Clin Radiol 1989; 40:325.
8. Ingle H, Nasim A, Bolia A, et al. Subintimal angioplasty of isolated infragenicular vessels in lower limb ischemia: long-term results. J Endovasc Ther 2002; 9:411–16.
9. Reekers JA, Bolia A. Percutaneous intentional extraluminal (subintimal) recanalization: how to do it yourself. Eur J Radiol 1998; 28:192–8.
10. Lipsitz EC, Ohki T, Veith FJ, et al. Does subintimal angioplasty have a role in the treatment of severe lower extremity ischemia? J Vasc Surg 2003; 37:386–91.
11. Nadal LL, Cynamon J, Lipsitz EC, Bolia A. Subintimal angioplasty for chronic arterial occlusions. Tech Vasc Interv Radiol 2004; 7:16–22.
12. Lipsitz EC, Veith FJ, Ohki T. The value of subintimal angioplasty in the management of critical lower extremity ischemia: failure is not always associated with a rethreatened limb. J Cardiovasc Surg (Torino) 2004; 45:231–7.
13. Dorrucci V. Treatment of superficial femoral artery occlusive disease. J Cardiovasc Surg (Torino) 2004; 45:193–201.
14. Colombo A, Mikhail GW, Michev I, et al. Treating chronic total occlusions using subintimal tracking and reentry: the STAR technique. Catheter Cardiovasc Interv 2005; 64:407–11; discussion 412.
15. Saketkhoo RR, Razavi MK, Padidar A, et al. Percutaneous bypass: subintimal recanalization of peripheral occlusive disease with IVUS guided luminal re-entry. Tech Vasc Interv Radiol 2004; 7:23–7.
16. Werner GS, Schwarz G, Prochnau D, et al. Paclitaxel-eluting stents for the treatment of chronic total coronary occlusions: a strategy of extensive lesion coverage with drug-eluting stents. Catheter Cardiovasc Interv 2006; 67:1–9.

6

Technical options for uncrossable lesions

Masahiko Ochiai

Appropriate balloon manipulation • Exchange of guide catheters or 'a child catheter in a mother' system • Anchoring • The Tornus crossing catheter • How to use the Tornus for the balloon uncrossable lesions • Case example with Tornus use • Countermeasures for failure of the Tornus • New wiring technique using the Tornus • Rotablator • Dilatation of the channel by the parallel wire technique

In recent years, difficulty in advancing the balloon often occurs after successfully crossing the lesion with a wire during percutaneous coronary intervention (PCI) for chronic total occlusion (CTO). Although the ability of balloons to pass through hard lesions has been improved owing to various device modifications, such as a smaller profile, they still fall behind the rapid advances in performance and technique that have occurred with CTO wires.[1-5] The frequency of such difficulties is thought to be considerably higher than several years ago. Although many old CTO lesions show extensive calcification,[6] it has become possible to advance a wire through such lesions, which used to be impenetrable.

My preference is to cross a CTO by manipulating the wire with the support of a microcatheter. After the wire has been passed, the microcatheter is removed by the Nanto method,[7] and then I usually try to advance a 1.5 mm single-operator exchange (SOE) balloon. If the lesion cannot be crossed, use of the following special methods should be taken into consideration. Like the parallel wire and the side-branch techniques, these methods are technically important in PCI for CTO. It is unwise to adhere to one particular strategy. Different techniques may be required for penetration of the proximal and distal fibrous caps, even in the same patient.

APPROPRIATE BALLOON MANIPULATION

First, the guide catheter is firmly engaged into the coronary artery to provide strong support. Then, the balloon is pushed against the lesion with alternating fine forward and backward movements. This procedure utilizes the physical principle that dynamic friction is smaller than static friction. Balloon passage is also promoted by deep inspiration, because the guide catheter and the balloon shaft are stretched.

If balloon passage cannot be achieved by this technique, the 1.5 mm balloon is pushed against the lesion as firmly as possible and then is inflated up to approximately 12 atm. The guide catheter is firmly engaged into the ostium of the coronary artery again. Immediately after deflation, the balloon should be further pushed into the lesion. If even a small part of the balloon tip becomes engaged into the lesion, it is expected that a small crack will be made in the hard lesion by balloon inflation. After the balloon has been inflated once, however, its crossing profile will be reduced. Therefore, if this technique results in failure, it will become more difficult for the balloon to cross the lesion. Although this technique will never be successful if there is no encroachment of the balloon tip into the lesion, it is impossible to judge the presence or absence of minor encroachment by fluoroscopy.

EXCHANGE OF GUIDE CATHETERS OR 'A CHILD IN A MOTHER' CATHETER SYSTEM

A guiding catheter can be exchanged into a different one, which provides stronger support, keeping the position of the wire in the coronary artery. This

(a)

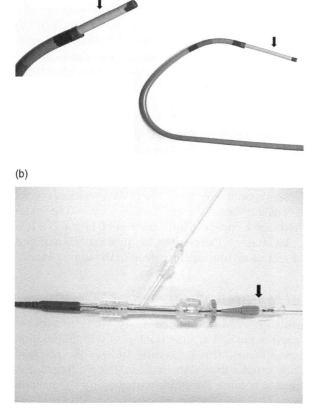

(b)

Figure 6.1 A 130 cm 5 Fr straight catheter (Terumo Corporation, Tokyo, Japan). It can be inserted across the Y-connector and advanced into the proximal part of the coronary artery.

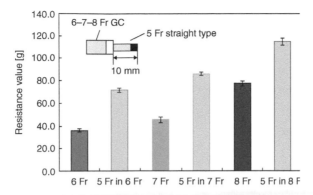

Figure 6.2 Measurement of the back-up support with 'a child catheter in a mother' system. The chart shows the back-up support of a JL4 guiding catheter in a glass model mimicking a human aorta and coronary artery. The resistance value was measured, when the guiding catheter dislodged from the ostium after pushing the wire and balloon into the coronary artery. When a 5 Fr catheter is put into a 6 Fr, the back-up support is stronger than that of a 7 Fr alone. Also, a 5 Fr in a 7 Fr catheter has stronger back-up support than that of an 8 Fr. GC, Guide catheter.

method is sometimes very effective. However, the wire may become dislodged occasionally before completion of the maneuver, resulting in complete failure. Therefore, for a CTO lesion, it is very important to select a guide catheter (at least 7 Fr) that provides strong support. If difficulty in advancing the balloon is expected, it is also recommended to insert a 65 cm iron metal sheath (Arrow International, Reading, PA) in advance. The support obtained with this sheath is approximately as strong as that obtained with a guide catheter that is 1 Fr larger in diameter.

Another way to enhance the back-up support much more conveniently and easily than by the exchange of guide catheters is to apply 'a child catheter in a mother' system.[8] A 130 cm 5 Fr straight catheter (Terumo Corporation, Tokyo, Japan) is deeply engaged into the proximal part of the target coronary artery across the Y-connector (Figure 6.1). A guide catheter with a diameter of 7 Fr or more (or a 6 Fr catheter with an inner diameter of ≥0.071 inch) can easily accept this 5 Fr straight catheter. If anchoring can be performed by using a balloon proximal to the CTO or in a branch vessel, deep engagement of the 5 Fr straight catheter can be achieved with more certainty. The support obtained by the 'a child catheter in a mother' system is approximately as strong as that achieved with a guide catheter that is 1 Fr larger in size (Figure 6.2).

ANCHORING

It is very convenient to perform anchoring using a branch vessel proximal to the CTO for enhancing back-up support.[9] At first, a 1.5 mm SOE balloon is inserted up to the occlusion. Then, a floppy wire is inserted into the branch vessel, and another SOE balloon for anchoring is advanced to the side branch and inflated to approximately 4–8 atm. Anchoring can also be done at the proximal part of the major vessel. After opening the Y-connector, while gently pulling back this anchoring balloon and the floppy wire with the left hand, the SOE balloon is advanced towards the occlusion with the right hand (Figure 6.3). Since the entire

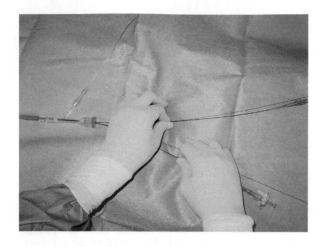

Figure 6.3 Maneuvers of anchoring. The penetrating balloon is advanced with the right hand while gently pulling the anchoring balloon and its wire with the left hand.

system (including the guide catheter) is fixed with the anchoring balloon, extremely strong support can be obtained. If the anchoring balloon comes out when it is difficult to advance the SOE balloon through the occlusion, the following countermeasures may be effective: (1) if the stenosis is located in a branch vessel, the anchoring balloon is inflated ahead of it or (2) another ('buddy') wire is placed between the anchoring balloon and the branch vessel to increase frictional resistance.

Complications with anchoring

Peculiar complications may occur during anchoring, as is the case with all PCI procedures.

Prolapse of the SOE balloon

When advancing the SOE balloon through the occlusion proves extremely difficult (e.g. when the lesion is located at the proximal left circumflex coronary artery [LCx]), the balloon shaft and the wire may prolapse toward the large side branch (e.g. left anterior descending artery [LAD]) and injure the vessel.

Pinhole rupture of the SOE balloon

Anchoring is performed to allow a balloon to pass through the occlusion with a severe superficial calcification. If there is a protrusion of the calcium, it may rupture the balloon. I have experienced two cases of balloon rupture, and the defect was a pinhole in both cases. It led to extravascular leakage of a small quantity of contrast medium in one patient, whereas intramural hematoma developed in the other.

THE TORNUS CROSSING CATHETER

The Tornus (Asahi Intec, Nagoya, Japan) crossing catheter is a special microcatheter for penetrating the hard lesions. It has a blunt tip (1 mm) that is mainly composed of platinum and eight bundles of stainless steel wire extend from the tip.

In Japan, the 2.1 Fr Tornus (diameter of the stainless steel wire = 0.12 mm, screw pitch = 1.1 mm) was released in March 2004[10] (Figure 6.4). The 2.6 Fr Tornus (diameter of the stainless steel wire = 0.18 mm, screw pitch = 1.7 mm) became available in January 2005 (see Figure 6.4). The 2.6 Fr Tornus shows superior transmission of torque and can be advanced more easily through a lesion to create a larger lumen. However, the 2.1 Fr Tornus is slightly better for following curved vessels.

Each of these catheters is designed so that the stainless steel wire acts like a screw against the vessel wall and is advanced manually by counterclockwise rotation. Actually, the tip (1 mm) of the Tornus is largely made of platinum. Although its profile is slightly larger than that of the 1.5 mm SOE balloon (Figure 6.5), it can pass through the balloon 'uncrossable' lesions because of

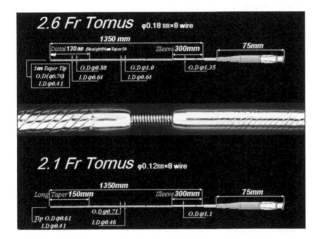

Figure 6.4 The 2.1 Fr and 2.6 Fr Tornus catheters.

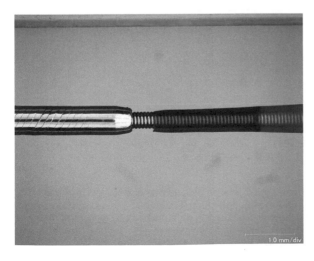

Figure 6.5 Comparison of the tips of the 2.6 Fr Tornus and 1.5 mm Maverick-2 Balloon (Boston Scientific, Maple Grove, MN). The left tip (silver) is Tornus 2.6 Fr and the right tip (red) is the Marverick-2 balloon.

two reasons: (1) the driving force generated by counterclockwise rotation against the vascular wall is very strong, and (2) the Tornus will not bend, unlike a polyamide balloon, because it is made of stainless steel (Figure 6.6). When optical coherence tomography was done after passing a 2.1 Fr Tornus through the occlusion, a 0.6–0.7 mm smooth lumen was observed. The incidence of dissection is much lower than for conventional balloon dilatation.

(a)

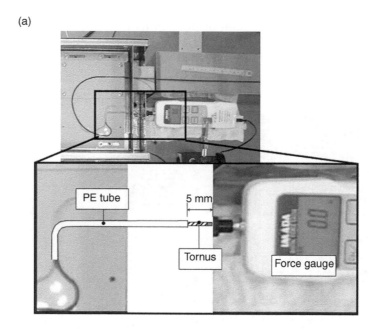

(b)

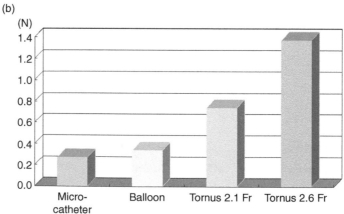

Figure 6.6 Comparison of the driving force in each crossing device. (a) Driving force was measured with a force gauge in a glass model mimicking a human aorta and coronary artery. (b) In a microcatheter and a balloon, their proximal parts were pushed and the largest load was measured at the gauge. In a Tornus 2.1 Fr and 2.6 Fr, they were rotated counterclockwise. The driving force of the Tornus was much larger than a microcatheter or a balloon. N = Newtons.

HOW TO USE THE TORNUS FOR THE BALLOON UNCROSSABLE LESIONS

When use of a Tornus is expected, a Y-connector with a hemostatic valve is attached in advance to ensure good torque transmission and prevent blood loss during its manipulation. I usually employ an OKAY Y-connector (Goodman, Nagoya, Japan). After an extension wire is attached to the stiff wire that is used to penetrate the CTO, the Tornus is inserted into the coronary artery via the guide catheter and is advanced to a point immediately proximal to the occlusion. The assistant should firmly fix the wire to prevent it from being pushed into the distal coronary artery during advancement of Tornus (Figure 6.7a).

The torquer is then firmly gripped with the fourth and fifth fingers of the right hand of the operator in order to prevent rotation of the wire together with the Tornus. The Tornus is advanced by counterclockwise rotation with the first to

(a)

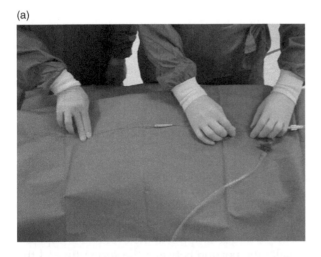

(b)

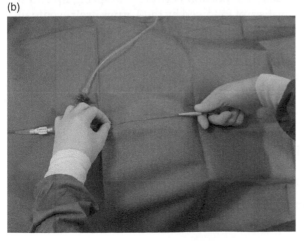

Figure 6.7 Manipulation of the Tornus, as described in the text.

third fingers of the right hand (Figure 6.7b). When the Tornus is being advanced, there is a risk of distal coronary artery perforation due to unexpected advancement or rotation of the stiff wire. If the lesion is very resistant to penetration, the guide catheter may fall off while all attention is concentrated on manipulating the Tornus. Therefore, it is important to select an adequate fluoroscopic view and magnification to allow clear recognition of both the guide catheter and wire tip.

To prevent disruption of the eight bundles of stainless steel wire inside the coronary artery, the Tornus is designed so that the wire bundles become disconnected at the stopper located at the hub against the excessive counterclockwise torque. The upper limits of counterclockwise rotation with its tip fixed are '40 times' in the 2.1 Fr Tornus and '20 times' in the 2.6 Fr Tornus. It might be considered that the tip is not fixed so long as the Tornus continues to advance through the CTO. However, caution must be exercised when it becomes stuck in the CTO and torque builds up. In this case, before the upper limit of the number of rotations is reached, the accumulated torque must be released by appropriately loosening your hold on the device.

If it is confirmed by fluoroscopy that the Tornus has obviously reached the distal coronary artery, the stiff wire for crossing the CTO can be removed. I prefer to replace the stiff wire by a floppy one, such as a Prowater (Asahi Intec), before the Tornus is removed. If the Tornus is used in a tortuous vessel, strong resistance can sometimes be felt when the stiff wire is pulled for exchange. In this case, the Tornus should be removed first and 1.5 SOE balloon crossing should be reattempted before wire replacement.

When the Tornus is being removed from a lesion, clockwise rotation should be applied under fluoroscopy. After replacing the stiff wire by a floppy wire, the Tornus can be removed more easily if the floppy wire is gently pushed against the distal coronary artery during clockwise rotation of the device. During clockwise rotation, it is mandatory to release accumulated torque before the upper limit (2.1 Fr Tornus – 40 revolutions, 2.6 Fr Tornus – 20 revolutions) as well. For structural reasons, the wire bundles of the Tornus are wringed by clockwise rotation. Therefore, if excessive clockwise torque is applied, the overload is imposed on a weak part of the wire (usually the portion between the spring tip and the shaft) and the wire bundles may disrupt followed by the Tornus itself eventually. The release of torque accumulated by clockwise rotation is slower than counterclockwise rotation because of the structure of the device, and requires more patience.

The Nanto method cannot be used for the Tornus when it is pulled out from the guide catheter. Instead, it must be pulled out under fluoroscopy with an extension or a 300 cm wire.

CASE EXAMPLE WITH TORNUS USE

The Tornus was effective in a 68-year-old male patient who underwent PCI for CTO at the LAD orifice. Contralateral angiography was performed using a microcatheter (Navicath, Terumo Corporation), which was inserted superselectively into the conus branch (Figure 6.8a). After a 7 Fr Brite-tip XB 3.5 (Cordis,

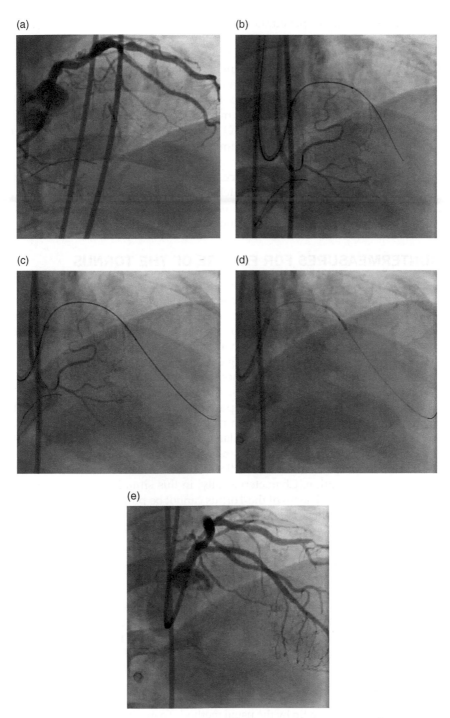

Figure 6.8 A patient in whom the balloon failed, but the 2.1 Fr Tornus was effective, as described in the text.

Miami, FL) was inserted, penetration of the lesion by a Confianza Pro (9 g) was attempted with the support of a microcatheter (Strider, Asahi Intec). Eventually, it was possible to pass through the CTO with a Confianza Pro 12 g (Figure 6.8b). Unfortunately, the CTO was balloon uncrossable and there was no side branch suitable for anchoring. The 2.1 Fr Tornus could pass through the CTO easily (Figure 6.8c). After the Confianza Pro 12 g was replaced by a Prowater, the Tornus was removed. Then, a 1.5–15 mm Maverick-2 balloon (Boston Scientific, Maple Grove, MN) could cross the CTO very easily (Figure 6.8d). An excellent dilatation of the CTO was obtained by implanting two stents until the ostium of the LAD (Figure 6.8e).

According to my personal experience, the success rate of the Tornus for the balloon-uncrossable CTO is approximately 85–90%.[11] After successful passage of a 2.1 Fr Tornus, a 1.5 mm balloon can usually cross the CTO. If a 2.6 Fr Tornus can cross the lesion, even a 2.0–2.5 mm balloon can be advanced frequently.

COUNTERMEASURES FOR FAILURE OF THE TORNUS

The failure of the Tornus consists of the following two situations.

First, the tip of the Tornus cannot be advanced at all, although marked accumulation of counterclockwise torque is noted. If the occlusion is extremely long and very hard, only a small amount of torque may be converted into driving force, which is not strong enough to advance its blunt tip through the lesion. We can restart counterclockwise rotation again after the accumulated counterclockwise torque is released. As a result, the Tornus can often be advanced slowly. However, the transmission of clockwise torque for its removal also tends to be very difficult in such lesions, which imposes some risk of wire disruption. If the tip cannot be advanced at all, although counterclockwise rotation is performed several times while releasing accumulated torque, I do not persist with this device and try a different modality or strategy instead.

Secondly, the Tornus continues to idle and cannot be advanced at all despite counterclockwise rotation. Characteristically, in this situation, accumulation of torque is not observed. The tip of the Tornus cannot be plunged into the lesion at all due to severe superficial calcium. Besides, any driving force cannot be generated despite counterclockwise rotation, because the part of the vascular wall in contact with the wire bundles of the Tornus has already been broken.

If the Tornus continues to idle and cannot be advanced at all, the following countermeasures should be taken. If this occurs near the distal fibrous cap of the occlusion, the stiff wire can be exchanged through the Tornus lumen into a Rotafloppy wire by the 'bare wire exchange' method. Then we can debulk the superficial calcium with a Rotablator. Actually, the success rate of the bare wire exchange method is extremely high near the distal cap. On the other hand, if this problem occurs near the proximal fibrous cap or in the middle of the CTO, it is difficult to apply the technique. I have obtained good results in two patients by plunging the distal tip of a 1.5 or 1.25 mm balloon into the Tornus-resistant lesion to make a small crack and then inserting the Tornus again. It is of course impossible to plunge the balloon tip by the usual method. To markedly enhance the back-up support, the anchor balloon technique or the 'a child catheter in a mother ' system should be applied in this situation.

NEW WIRING TECHNIQUE USING THE TORNUS

The driving force of the Tornus is much stronger than that of a balloon provided that its tip can be plunged into the CTO. Since the driving force is generated by the screwing effect, the Tornus does not require much support. Furthermore, it has a tip marker, unlike a 1.5 mm over-the-wire (OTW) balloon, so its position can be confirmed clearly. The lumen obtained with a Tornus is also smoother than that achieved with a balloon, which tends to cause dissection. I have tried four novel strategies so far with this device, as follows (with case examples).[5,11]

Enhancement of back-up support for wire cross

If even the dedicated stiff wire for a CTO cannot be advanced at all inside the occlusion, the Tornus can be engaged forcefully from the proximal end of the CTO. It fixes against the CTO and provides strong back-up support for wiring. The operator should be confident that the wire is located in the true lumen before engagement of the Tornus.

A 46-year-old man underwent retry of PCI for mid-LAD CTO due to occlusion of a stent that had been implanted 4 years previously (Figure 6.9a). After inserting a 7 Fr Heart-rail BL 3.5 (Terumo Corporation), a Confianza Pro (9 g) and then a Confianza Pro 12 g were tried with the support of a microcatheter (Navicath, Terumo Corporation). However, there was very hard tissue at a certain point located several millimeters distal from the proximal edge of the CTO, so the tip of these wires deviated from the correct course. Since it was also impossible to advance a Navicath into the CTO (Figure 6.9b), a 2.1 Fr Tornus was then engaged at the proximal part of the CTO (Figure 6.9c). The back-up support for wiring was enhanced dramatically, and a Confianza Pro 12 g wire could be advanced further (Figure 6.9d). After the CTO was crossed by the Confianza Pro 12 g, the 2.1 Fr Tornus could be passed through easily. Then predilatation was carried out with 1.5 and 2.5 mm balloons, after which three stents were implanted (Figure 6.9e).

Wire exchange inside the CTO

Even after successful penetration of the very hard part of the CTO by a stiff wire such as Confianza Pro, further advancement of the wire may be blocked if the distal coronary artery is so tortuous. In a typical case, although a so-called 'middle island' is secured, it is difficult to advance the stiff wire distal to the island, if the distal vessel beyond the island has a tiny and tortuous antegrade microchannel. The stiff wire is not suitable to follow this kind of antegrade microchannel. In the conventional method, after penetration of the CTO by a 1.5 mm OTW balloon, the wire is replaced with a more slippery one. However, since the Confianza Pro has not reached the distal coronary artery, back-up support for the OTW balloon is insufficient and it sometimes fails to cross the CTO. Furthermore, since the marker of the OTW balloon is usually located at its center, the position of the balloon tip cannot be recognized by fluoroscopy, which makes this procedure more challenging. The Tornus is highly effective under these conditions.

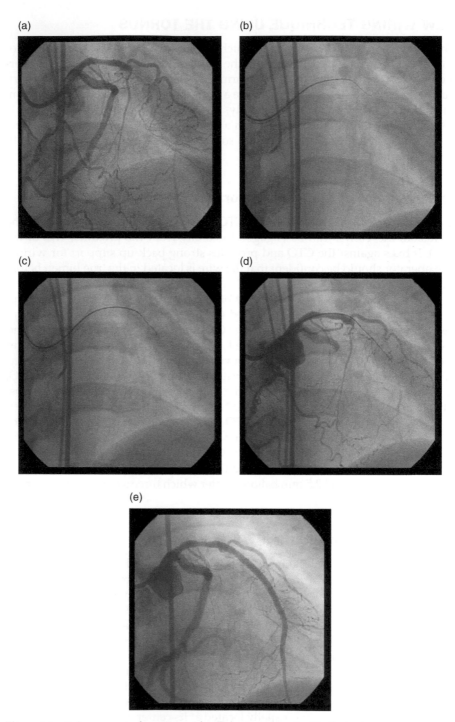

Figure 6.9   Enhancement of support with a Tornus, as described in the text.

A 68-year-old man underwent PCI for a CTO at the ostium of the LAD due to anteroseptal myocardial infarction that had occurred 7 years ago (Figure 6.10a). The CTO was extremely long (Figure 6.10b), good collateral was supplied from the septal branches, and a 'middle island' was clearly noted (single arrow). The antegrade blood flow from the 'middle island' seemed to compete with the retrograde blood flow from epicardial collaterals around the apex to form a functional total occlusion (double arrow), although it was difficult to identify on the static image. Although the 'middle island' was reached with a Confianza Pro (9 g) (Figure 6.10c), it could not follow the distal tortuous microchannel. Therefore, a 2.1 Fr Tornus was advanced to the 'middle island,' while the Confianza Pro was kept in the septal branch (Figure 6.10d). Then the Confianza Pro was removed (Figure 6.10e) and replaced by a Fielder, a plastic and hydrophilic-coated wire (Asahi Intec). The Fielder could easily follow the microchannel and be advanced into the distal vessel (Figure 6.10f). After predilatation, three stents were implanted (Figure 6.10g).

Application to the side-branch technique

A 1.5 mm balloon is generally used for the side-branch technique. However, there is always a risk of dissection by balloon dilatation, which will lead to failure of the procedure. The incidence of dissection is rare in the Tonus, which can also make some connection between the side branch and the main vessel. The 2.6 Fr Tornus is more preferable for this purpose, because it can create a larger lumen.

A 54-year-old man underwent PCI for a mid-LAD CTO located at the origin of the second diagonal branch (Figure 6.11a). After inserting an 8 Fr Mach 1 FCL 4.0 (Boston Scientific), penetration was started using a Confianza Pro (9 g) with the support of a microcatheter (Navicath, Terumo Corporation). Finally, the second diagonal was penetrated by the parallel wire technique using a Confianza Pro 12g (Figure 6.11b). Then the 2.6 Fr Tornus was advanced to the diagonal, and the wire was replaced by a Prowater (Figure 6.11c). After removing the Tornus, a floppy wire (Runthrough NS, Terumo Corporation) was advanced with the support of Navicath. Since the CTO itself had been completely penetrated by the Tornus and some connection was created between the diagonal and the LAD, the floppy wire could be easily advanced into the lumen of the LAD (Figure 6.11d). After predilatation, three stents were implanted and kissing dilatation was performed at the left main coronary artery (Figure 6.11e).

Reentry into the distal coronary artery from the subintimal space

If the true lumen cannot be obtained despite repeated parallel wire technique and the wire can be advanced close to the proximal end of the distal coronary artery, the Tornus can be advanced over the wire, whose tip is still in the subintimal space. After the torque transmission and the back-up support is enhanced by the advancement of the Tornus, we can manipulate the wire again to create a reentry into the true lumen.

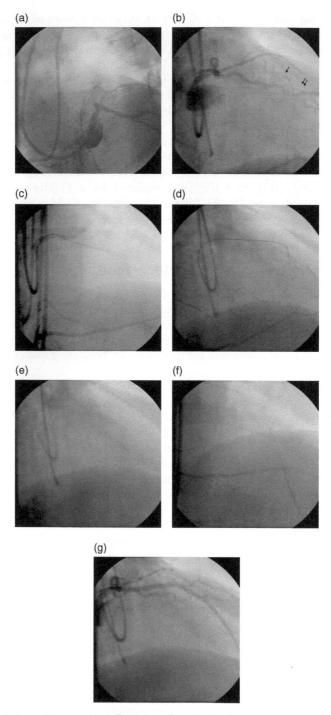

Figure 6.10   Wire exchange using a Tornus, as described in the text.

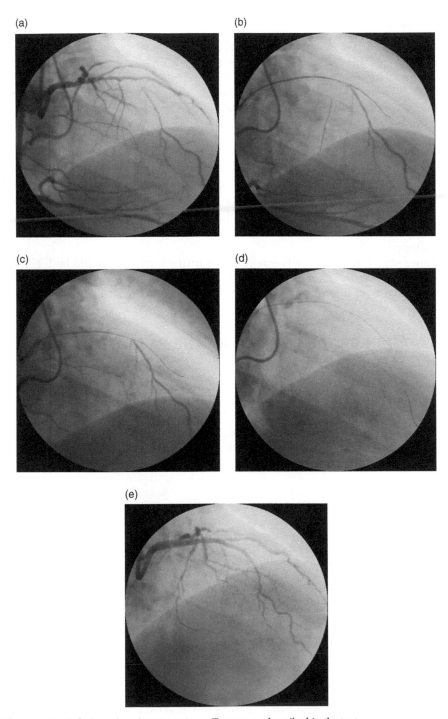

Figure 6.11   Side-branch technique using a Tornus, as described in the text.

ROTABLATOR

The Rotablator is very effective in debulking superficial calcification of balloon-uncrossable CTO. First, the stiff wire that has crossed the CTO should be exchanged for a Rotafloppy using the 'bare wire exchange' method. The most reliable 1.5 mm OTW balloon is advanced as far as possible. When it stops, the screw of the Y-connector is tightened to fix the balloon so that it does not come out of the guide catheter. Then, the stiff wire is pulled out completely, and the CTO should be recrossed by the Rotafloppy. If the Rotafloppy fails to recross the CTO, the procedure results in failure. However, the success rate of the 'bare wire exchange' method is extremely high provided that the balloon was blocked near the distal fibrous cap. In such a balloon-uncrossable part of the CTO, the possibility of the wire entering the subintimal space is low, owing to circumferential superficial calcification. Furthermore, since the stiff wire has already penetrated the CTO, at least a small lumen is already available, which can be followed by the Rotafloppy.

Since severe calcification is expected, the initial burr size should be 1.25 mm, even when the reference vessel diameter is large. Repeated rapid pecking movement of the burr for several seconds at the maximum speed is preferred in my current practice.

DILATATION OF THE CHANNEL BY THE PARALLEL WIRE TECHNIQUE

The wire that has crossed the CTO is left in situ, while another stiff wire is inserted parallel to it and advanced by repeated pushing and pulling so that it is entangled with the first wire and dilates the lumen. For this purpose, a Miraclebros 12g is the best choice. If a successful lesion cross is not achieved with the Miraclebros 12g, it is sometimes worthwhile to intentionally manipulate the wire in the subintimal space so that the calcified tissue is broken down.

REFERENCES

1. Stone GW, Kandzari DE, Mehran R et al. Percutaneous recanalization of chronically occluded coronary arteries: consensus document: part I. Circulation 2005; 112:2364–72.
2. Stone GW, Reifart NJ, Moussa I, et al. Percutaneous recanalization of chronically occluded coronary arteries: consensus document: Part II. Circulation 2005; 112:2530–7.
3. Stone GW, Colombo A, Teirstein P, et al. Percutaneous recanalization of chronically occluded coronary arteries: procedural techniques, devices and results. Catheter Cardiovasc Interv 2005; 66:217–36.
4. Ochiai M, Ashida K, Araki H, et al. The latest wire technique for chronic total occlusions. Ital Heart J 2005; 6:489–93.
5. Ochiai M. Logical Analysis and Re-construction of Percutaneous Coronary Intervention. Tokyo: Chugai Igaku; 2005. [in Japanese]
6. Fujii K, Ochiai M, Mintz GS, et al. Procedural implications of intravascular ultrasound morphologic features of chronic total coronary occlusion. Am J Cardiol 2006; 97:1455–62.
7. Nanto S, Ohara T, Shimonagata T, Hori M, Kubori S. A technique for exchanging a PTCA balloon catheter over a regular-length guidewire. Cathet Cardiovasc Diagn 1994; 23:341–6.
8. Takahashi S, Saito S, Tanaka S, et al. New method to increase a backup support of a 6 French guiding coronary catheter. Catheter Cardiovasc Intervent 2004; 63:452–6.

9. Fujita S, Tamai H, Kyo E, et al. New technique for superior guiding catheter support during advancement of a balloon in coronary angioplasty: the anchor technique. Catheter Cardiovasc Interv 2003; 59:484–8.

10. Tsuchikane E, Katoh O, Shimogami M, et al. First clinical experience of a novel penetration catheter for patients with severe coronary artery stenosis. Catheter Cardiovasc Interv 2005; 65:368–73.

11. Ochiai M, Ashida K, Araki H, Ogata N, Obara C. Impact of Tornus™ vascular microcatheter in chronic total occlusion. Am J Cardiol 2005; 96:162H.

7

Rotational atherectomy

Mark Reisman

Mechanism of action • Clinical results in chronic total occlusions • Case examples • Conclusion

Rotational atherectomy (RA) has been well described as a device effective in plaque modification that specifically increases vessel compliance and permits the transit of balloons and stents in heavily calcified arteries, despite a demonstrated increased minimal luminal diameter on the final angiogram when stenting is performed with adjunctive RA, this has not been translated into a lower restenosis rate, and thus the device has been primarily relegated to improving acute outcomes and procedural success.

The role of RA in chronic total occlusions (CTOs) is ultimately based on the success of crossing the lesion with the guidewire. Once achieved, and the true lumen is accessed, RA can facilitate, via debulking, the crossing of balloons and stents, and in this era, primarily drug-eluting stents, to optimize the final result. The technical characteristics of the device are described in Figure 7.1.

MECHANISMS OF ACTION

Orthogonal displacement of friction

Orthogonal displacement of friction describes the physical property of a rotating device producing decreased frictional forces in the plane perpendicular to the spinning vector, i.e. in the longitundinal plane for the advancing burr. An example of this effect is the removal of a cork from a wine bottle or the removal of a ring from one's finger; it is done much easier when rotating while withdrawing the object due to the reduced frictional forces.

This salutary effect allows the burr to negotiate the most tortuous vessels and those vessels that are very small in caliber due to disease, as would be seen in CTOs.

Differential cutting

Differential cutting, the hallmark of the RA system, refers to the ability of the burr to ablate or 'sand' inelastic material while sparing elastic tissue. The elastic

(a)

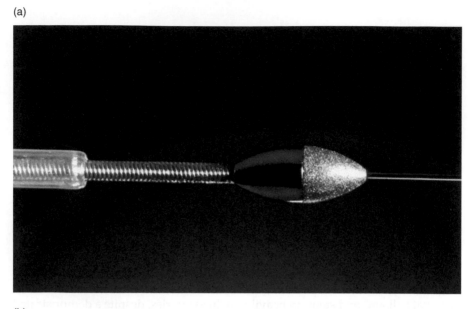

(b)

Console

Rotational speed display (tachometer)

Procedure timer

Turbine pressure gauge (delivered to advancer)

Reset button

Event timer

Turbine pressure control knob (adjusts rpm)

Advancer fiberoptic tachometer connector

Power switch

Dynaglide™ connector

Advancer turbine (pneumatic) connector

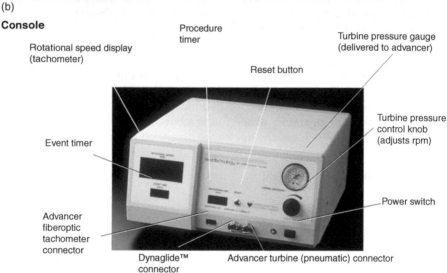

Figure 7.1 The Rotablator device: (a) burr and wire and (b) console.

(normal) tissue simply deflects from the advancing burr, while the more inelastic tissue (atherosclerotic plaque) is treated with rotational atherectomy. An example is shaving. The inelastic whiskers are removed by the razor, while the skin deflects away from the blade.

This physical property of the burr thus would be very helpful in treating CTOs since the majority of them have elements of calcium and fibrocalcific disease.[1] This would result in decreased vessel compliance and thus would help the advancement of balloons and stents and would have a beneficial impact on the final minimal lumen diameter (MLD) of the vessel post stenting.[2]

Procedure

The initial crossing of the CTO should be carried out in the safest and most efficacious way in order to maximally assure the positioning in the true lumen throughout. Once the guidewire is placed distally, the challenge at times may be to exchange for a rotawire. This can be done with a low-profile balloon or a number of catheter exchange devices that are available on the market.

Depending on the anatomy, one can exchange for either the RotaWire Floppy or the RotaWire Extra Support, with the floppy wire being advantageous in tortuous vessels and the extrasupport wire helpful at times for improved lesion purchase or advancing the device to the lesion site. Often, owing to the extensive disease, it is necessary to activate the device proximal to the treatment site to take advantage of the reduced friction of the spinning burr. Once the burr is positioned proximal to the site, a contrast injection to verify that there is flow around the burr is critical so that the burr is not activated in a constrained segment. This can lead to significant heat generation and possible dissection. The burr speed should be approximately 150 000 rpm, and a technique of gentle advancement and retraction with occasional contrast dye injections is optimal. Using the smaller burrs (1.25 mm, 1.5 mm) an abrupt deceleration when advancing slowly should be of concern that the wire is subintimal; the burr should be withdrawn and an angiogram performed to be certain that no significant dissection or perforation has occurred. In the absence of antegrade flow after wire placement, it is generally recommended to initiate treatment with a 1.25 mm burr. If the device is being applied in a non-compliant segment that is undilatable (with a lumen demonstrated angiographically), then it is acceptable to start with a larger device. Rotational atherectomy can be performed after attempted percutaneous transluminal coronary angioplasty (PTCA) of an undilatable segment as long as there is no evidence of significant dissection or dye staining. Since the goal is lesion modification to alter compliance, the burr:artery ratio will rarely need to exceed 0.7. Once increased vessel compliance has been achieved as well as access to the lesion site for stents, the guidewire is generally exchanged for a more preferable 'stent wire' and the remainder of the procedure is completed.

CLINICAL RESULTS IN CHRONIC TOTAL OCCLUSIONS

Tsuchikane et al[3] reported a series of patients with CTO treated with RA (Rotablator, Boston Scientific/Scimed, Inc., Maple Grove, MN) followed by bare metal stent implantation. This study was a non-randomized retrospective comparison with a group of patients treated with stenting alone prior to the advent of RA. In the Rotablator group, RA was performed only if the operator was convinced that the guidewire was in the true lumen; a total of 50 patients were recanalized and treated with RA, restoring TIMI (Thrombolysis in Myocardial Infarction) grade 3 antegrade flow in all the cases. No major adverse events occurred; only one non-Q wave myocardial infarction (MI) was observed (2%). Statistically significant differences were found in both the post-procedure and the 6-month follow-up lumen dimensions favoring the group treated with RA compared with the group treated with stenting alone. Angiographic follow-up was obtained in 96% (in 48 of 50 patients) at 6 months; restenosis occurred in 29% of the patients treated with RA plus stenting compared with 52% in the group treated with stenting alone ($p = 0.0061$). By multivariate regression analysis, predictors of restenosis were pre-procedural lesion length, reference vessel diameter, and the application of RA.

In another early study, Dietz et al[4] studied 106 symptomatic patients who had 67 significant stenoses and 46 chronic occlusions. Rotational ablation could not be used in 16 chronic occlusions because of inability to cross the lesion and position the RA guidewire in the distal lumen. Initial angiographic and clinical success by rotational ablation was achieved in 18 chronic occlusions (39% of total, 56% of those treated with RA). Specifically, in the 30 chronic occlusions treated by rotational ablation, the angiographic diameter stenoses were reduced to 38% (18%). There were no procedural deaths and two patients (2%) underwent emergency coronary artery bypass grafting. Combined use of RA and balloon angioplasty was feasible and is necessary in about half of all procedures, because the lumen created by the biggest burr is too small. At 6 months, angiographic restenosis was evident in 14 of the 24 (58%) of chronic occlusions that were followed-up. Although no transmural infarction occurred, there were five (6%) non-Q-wave infarctions (two embolic side-branch occlusions, two subacute occlusions, and one acute occlusion). Severe, refractory coronary artery spasm was provoked in seven cases (8%).

Ho et al[5] reported the combination of the Frontrunner and RA in difficult CTO cases. This encountered two technical challenges: the inability of the balloon catheter to cross the CTO, and the inability to recross the occlusion with the less steerable RotaWire. This rather extreme example indicates that, when tackling difficult CTOs, a comprehensive strategy that encompasses multiple devices and technologies can enable ultimate procedural success.

CASE EXAMPLES

In the first case (Figure 7.2), a 58-year-old male presented with a CTO of a left anterior descending artery (LAD) segment that had been treated with a bare metal stent 2 years earlier. After an initial attempt at opening this CTO failed due to inability to cross with the guidewire, the patient was referred for a second attempt.

In Figure 7.2a, bilateral contrast injections (from both left and right coronary catheters) demonstrated CTO of the proximal LAD stent segment of the vessel. The CTO appears to extend proximal and distal to the stent.

Using a Miraclebros 6.0g guidewire (Figure 7.2b), the lesion was crossed and the distal vessel was able to be negotiated. Due to the constraining CTO, it was difficult to manipulate this wire distally, and judicious care was taken not to disrupt the distal vessel with the stiff guidewire.

Multiple attempts to exchange the guidewire failed due to inability to cross the lesion with several low-profile balloons, end-hole exchange catheters, and the Tornus catheter. Attempts were made to treat the vessel with the excimer laser, but this device was unable to cross the lesion. The only catheter to cross the lesion was the Excelsior catheter (Figure 7.2c). Despite exchanging for heavyweight

(a)

(b)

(c)

(d)

(e)

(f)

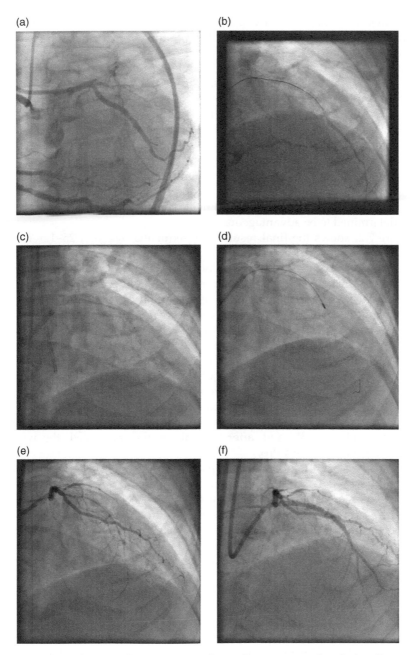

Figure 7.2 Recanalization of a left anterior descending artery total occlusion. See text for step-by-step technical details.

guidewires, including Choice Extrasupport and Grand Slam, we were still unable to cross the lesion with a balloon catheter. We then exchanged for a Rota Extra Support guidewire (0.009 inch shaft with 0.014 inch radiopaque tip).

Owing to the difficulties in crossing with low-profile systems and the lack of antegrade flow, the initial burr size was a 1.25 mm device (Figure 7.2d). This device has the lowest torque and optimal feedback/responsiveness. Therefore, if the guidewire was subintimal or behind a strut, a significant deceleration would occur with limited heat generation and lower probability for an adverse event such as perforation.

The typical appearance of the vessel after use of a small 1.25 mm burr is a narrow, smooth pilot lumen with limited antegrade flow (Figure 7.2e). At times it is not possible to visualize antegrade flow due to brisk retrograde collaterals or vasospasm after treatment. This should not deter further incremental burr usage if it is determined to be advantageous.

Figure 7.2f shows the final result after sequential use of 1.25–1.5–1.75 mm burrs and implantation of a 3.0 × 3 mm drug-eluting stent. In spite of the ablation, one can still observe incomplete expansion of the proximal stent. The distal vessel is somewhat attenuated distally secondary to excellent retrograde flow from the mature collaterals originating from the right coronary artery (RCA).

In the other case (Figure 7.3), a 51-year-old male with subtotal occlusion of a saphenous vein graft (SVG) to the RCA and an occluded native RCA is discussed. An earlier attempt to place a filter distal to the bulky SVG lesion was unsuccessful and the patient was referred for an attempt to open the native coronary CTO. A left anterior oblique view with dual injections from a catheter positioned at the ostium of the vein graft and the right coronary guide demonstrated severe stenosis in the distal SVG and the occluded proximal native RCA (Figure 7.3a).

Initial progress was made by the Prowater wire with a Voyager 1.5 mm balloon for support (Figure 7.3b) and, after the balloon was advanced, the wire was exchanged for a Confianza Pro.

After successful crossing of this complex CTO, an attempt was made to inflate a 2.5 mm balloon at 18 atm pressure at the proximal RCA segment; however, balloon expansion was impossible (Figure 7.3c).

Figure 7.3d shows the vessel after treatment with a 1.5 mm burr at 150 000 rpm. There were minimal decelerations when crossing the lesion. Subsequently, the same 2.5 mm balloon was now able to be fully expanded at 8 atm (Figure 7.3e). The final result post-stenting with excellent appearance of the mid section of the vessel is shown in Figure 7.3f; 2.5 mm Taxus stents were placed with 3.0 mm balloon post-dilatation.

CONCLUSION

Utilization of RA can be invaluable in certain CTO cases with very long and hard or uncrossable lesions. Innovative approaches need to be employed in order to safely place the special Rotablator wire in the distal lumen. Following this achievement, a small-size burr and a careful technique can debulk and modify the lesion compliance before the decision of further ablation or balloon inflation and, ultimately stent implantation, are undertaken.

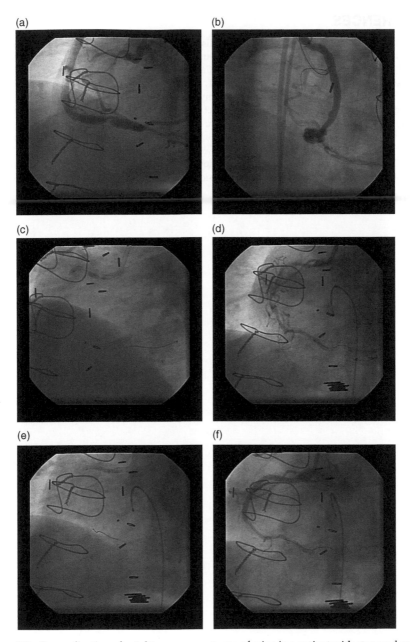

Figure 7.3 Recanalization of a right coronary artery occlusion in a patient with stenosed saphenous vein graft to this arterial territory. See text for step-by-step technical details.

REFERENCES

1. Srivatsa SS, Edwards WD, Boos CM, et al. Histologic correlates of angiographic chronic total coronary artery occlusions: influence of occlusion duration on neovascular channel patterns and intimal plaque composition. J Am Coll Cardiol 1997; 29:955-63.
2. Reisman M, Harms V, Whitlow P, Feldman T, Fortuna R, Buchbinder M. Comparison of early and recent results with rotational atherectomy. J Am Coll Cardiol 1997; 29(2):353-7.
3. Tsuchikane E, Otsuji S, Awata N, et al. Impact of pre-stent plaque debulking for chronic coronary total occlusions on restenosis reduction. J Invasive Cardiol 2001; 13(8):584-9.
4. Dietz U, Erbel R, Rupprecht HJ, Weidmann S, Meyer J. High-frequency rotational ablation: an alternative in treating coronary artery stenoses and occlusions. Br Heart J 1993; 70(4): 327-36.
5. Ho PC, Leung C, Chan S. Blunt microdissection and rotational atherectomy: an effective combination for the resistant chronic total occlusion. J Invasive Cardiol 2006; 18(9):E246-9.

8

Role of the CROSSER Catheter

Mark Reisman

Therapeutic ultrasound • Crosser Catheter • Case presentations • Clinical studies

Crossing chronic total occlusions (CTOs) continues to present a challenge for coronary and peripheral interventionalists. Limited imaging capabilities of the gap segment, identification of the true lumen, and the lack of guidewire responsiveness when positioned in a dense fibrocalcific milieu are all factors that contribute to this clinical challenge. In addition, current CTO crossing technologies, such as guidewires, require excessive procedure times associated with high contrast loads and significant radiation exposure to both the operator and the patient.

New CTO crossing technology would be more attractive if these issues could be addressed, as well as limiting complications in these complex lesions. A premium has therefore been placed on interventional devices that would be able to quickly and safely cross CTOs. One type of technology that has been evaluated as an energy source to facilitate recanalization of CTOs is therapeutic ultrasound.

THERAPEUTIC ULTRASOUND

Physical properties of ultrasound such as mechanical fragmentation, photo-acoustic cavitation, and microstreaming have generated interest for use in vascular occlusions[1-3] for quite a while. In-vivo and in-vitro studies have indicated that therapeutic ultrasound is not harmful to endothelial and smooth muscle cells,[4] promotes vasodilation, and most particles embolized are under 10 μm in diameter.[5]

These actions can be mediated as follows:

- Mechanical fragmentation occurs when the catheter acts as a vibrational jackhammer to disrupt the occlusion physically.
- Microbubbles form within the occlusion when subjected to ultrasound energy with a frequency of 5–17 MHz, and ensuing cavitation occurs as the bubbles expand/explode.
- Microstreaming is a secondary motion between differential shear–stress areas, due to aggregates of oscillating bubbles that increase shear stress and can break local vessel wall structures.

- Thermal effects from ultrasound energy (beyond the safety limit of 1°C) can potentially damage the vascular wall. The thermal effect can be desirable to break the substance of the occlusion, or can be minimized by active saline flush (cooling effect).

The first human clinical studies performed using therapeutic ultrasound as a tool for opening CTOs used the 20 kHz Sonicross system (Advanced Cardiovascular Systems, Santa Clara, CA). Procedural success was obtained in six of the 14 patients (43%). Complications included two localized perforations and four non-flow-limiting dissections.[6,7] The high device profile, relative shaft inflexibility, and procedural complexity all limited further development of this system.

These limitations of the first-generation device were addressed by the CROSSER Catheter (FlowCardia, Inc., Sunnyvale, CA). The CROSSER Catheter offers a different approach that allows the blunt catheter tip to present itself to the proximal cap, and high-frequency vibrational energy to be used to proceed through the blockage. Because of the relatively low force placed on the vessel and the device design, the potential may be for incremental results over the presently available technology while maintaining or improving procedural safety.

CROSSER CATHETER

Design of the CROSSER Catheter

This catheter system consists of reusable electronics (generator and transducer) and the single-use CROSSER Catheter (Figures 8.1 and 8.2). The CROSSER Catheter is connected to the electronics by attaching the proximal hub of the CROSSER to the distal end of the transducer. The generator converts AC line power into high-frequency current. This current is then delivered to piezoelectric crystals contained within the transducer, resulting in crystal expansion and contraction. The transducer horn amplifies the rapid crystal expansion and contraction, propagating high-frequency mechanical vibrations down a nitinol core wire to the stainless steel tip of the CROSSER Catheter at approximately 20 kHz or 20 000 cycles per second. The monorail device can be loaded onto a conventional guidewire system in order to bring the device to the totally occluded segment in the artery.

Mechanism of action

Mechanical impact and cavitation are two active methods for CTO recanalization using the CROSSER Catheter system.

Mechanical impact

The tip of the CROSSER Catheter mechanically vibrates against the face of the CTO at 20 000 cycles per second (20 kHz) at a stroke depth of approximately 20 μm. This high-frequency, low-amplitude longitudinal stroke pulverizes the CTO by mechanical impact and creates a channel through the CTO.

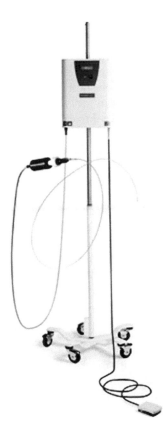

Figure 8.1   The FlowCardia CROSSER system includes the CROSSER Catheter and the console and foot pedal.

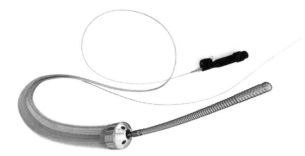

Figure 8.2   Close-up view of the tip of the CROSSER Catheter. This catheter transmits high-frequency vibrations at 20 000 cycles per second to the tip of the catheter. Its low profile enables access to TOs even in tortuous anatomy, and the monorail design allows alternation between CROSSER and standard guidewire techniques.

Cavitation

In addition to the direct mechanical ablation, high-frequency vibration can create vapor-filled microbubbles in the fluid (blood and saline) at the tip of the CROSSER Catheter. As the CROSSER Catheter is activated, these microbubbles expand and implode, producing liquid jets that can break the molecular bonds and erode the solid surface of the CTO.

It is hypothesized that the selective penetration of plaque with this catheter is dependent on the difference in elasticity between the atherosclerotic plaque and the adjacent media. Collagen, the major determinant of tissue elasticity, is abundant in the media of muscular arteries, whereas the collagen in atherosclerotic plaque is abnormal, making the elasticity of plaque significantly lower than that of the media. When vibrational energy is applied, a given level of energy causes more deformation and a greater disintegrative effect on the less elastic atherosclerotic plaque, as opposed to the more elastic arterial wall. High-frequency vibrational recanalization can cause some concern regarding unwanted impact on the vessel. One side effect is the local heating of tissues resulting from the dissipation of the catheter's mechanical energy. However, this has yet to become a clinically relevant concern with the CROSSER system, since 95% of this heating occurs at the proximal end of the catheter, which is outside the body. This fact, together with continuous saline irrigation at a flow rate of 18 ml/min, allows local heating at the catheter tip to be maintained at <1°C higher than normal.

Procedure/technique

Initial clinical experience with the CROSSER Catheter was reserved for the recalcitrant CTO lesions that could not be crossed with conventional guidewire systems as part of the European clinical trial and then in the US FACTOR (FlowCardia's Approach to Chronic Total Occlusion Recanalization) study. As experience has been gained with the system, certain caveats that allow for optimal performance of the system have been appreciated.

The monorail CROSSER Catheter is advanced to the totally occluded vessel over a conventional coronary guidewire. Guide catheter support is critical in order to get adequate pressure/engagement of the proximal cap of the CTO. This can be achieved at times with 6 Fr guide catheter systems and standard curves, but often benefits from larger (7–8 Fr) and more complex guide catheter shapes that maximize support. Prior to advancing the CROSSER Catheter, attempts had been made with guidewires; thus, it was not unusual for an entrance to the lesion or penetration to the lesion to have been accomplished. Theoretically, this had positive and negative impacts on overall success. It was beneficial in that it allowed an access point into the occlusion. However, if the guidewire had gone subintimal, it may result in a large dissection plane and the catheter would most likely become dedicated to the track created. Another benefit of having the guidewire penetrating into the lesion is based on the blunt tip of the catheter. The CROSSER Catheter will typically follow the path of least resistance and, if there is a side branch at the face of the CTO orientated in an unfavorable angle, it is often difficult to telescope the device into the CTO, away from the side branch. By positioning the guidewire into the occlusion, the CROSSER Catheter can be delivered over the guidewire directly, to engage the occlusion.

Once positioned at the CTO, we then withdraw the guidewire back into the monorail lumen and activate the device by stepping on a small foot pedal. The CROSSER Catheter is guided independently, and moves antegrade as the vibrational energy creates a path for advancement.

Gentle, forward pressure is recommended as the optimal strategy for advancing the catheter during activation. Once progress had been achieved, attempts to advance the guidewire into the true lumen of the vessel distal to the CTO are made. The use of bilateral injections is suggested to optimize visualization of the coronary anatomy Once the operator has navigated through the total occlusion, conventional percutaneous transluminal coronary angioplasty (PTCA) or other technologies followed by stents were usually performed.

CASE PRESENTATIONS

The first case (Figure 8.3) discusses a CTO of the left anterior descending artery of a 66-year-old man who underwent previous recanalization attempts.

In Figure 8.3a, a left anterior oblique caudal view with bilateral injections indicates the occlusion site to be just beyond the takeoff of a moderately sized diagonal branch. The distal vessel is seen clearly via right to left collaterals, with an occlusion segment of approximately 25 mm.

After making minimal progress with the Miracle 3 guidewire, and since the segment appeared to be relatively straight, the Confianza Pro guidewire was chosen (Figure 8.3b, right anterior oblique cranial view). The guidewire exchange and support was performed with a 1.5 × 9 mm Maverick balloon. At this point, we anticipated going to the Flocardia CROSSER system, since the guidewire attempt exceeded 10 minutes of fluoroscopic time and thus fulfilled the criteria for the protocol. The proximal cap has been penetrated and in multiple orthogonal views it appeared that the guidewire was 'lined up' with the distal vessel. Penetration of the proximal cap when a side branch is at the entry point of the CTO increases the likelihood the device will advance into the lesion as opposed to the side branch.

In Figure 8.3c, a left anterior oblique caudal view of the guidewire position raised concern of a potential subintimal orientation. Therefore, further advancement of the guidewire was not pursued. The CROSSER device would be taken to the point of achieving engagement of the cap, but not the full distance that the guidewire had traversed.

In Figure 8.3d (right anterior oblique cranial view), the CROSSER catheter was advanced into the lesion and the guidewire was withdrawn a few millimeters within the distal tip of the device. Once in this position, the flush was turned on, the foot pedal was depressed, the device was activated, and the device was then slowly advanced in a constant forward motion with occasional contrast injections.

The FlowCardia CROSSER device successfully crossed the lesion and the distal cap, and at that point successful distal placement of the guidewire was able to be achieved without resistance (Figure 8.3e). In general, attempts can be made to exit the guidewire from the device during the advancement into the total occlusion; if resistance is felt, then withdraw back into the CROSSER Catheter, until the distal cap is reached. During the treatment of long segments it is recommended to do orthogonal injections (bilateral) to make certain the catheter is tracking in the appropriate vector/direction of the treated vessel.

The final result after placement of two drug-eluting stents, with continued patency of the diagonal artery and an excellent angiographic result, is shown in Figure 8.3f.

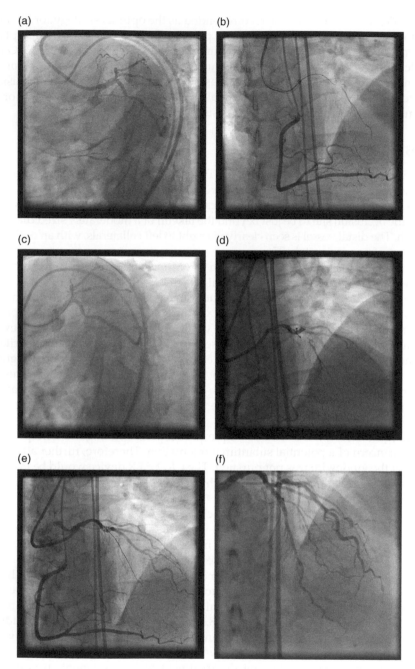

Figure 8.3   Recanalization of a left anterior descending artery using dual injection technique and the CROSSER catheter. See text for step–by–step details.

The other case (Figure 8.4) describes a 72-year-old-female with previous unsuccessful attempts to treat a right coronary artery (RCA) CTO that was referred for treatment with the FlowCardia CROSSER system.

Angiography with bilateral injections demonstrated a collateral flow pattern to the mid-RCA CTO: both intracoronary antegrade collaterals as well as retrograde from the left anterior descending artery (Figure 8.4a).

A right anterior oblique projection demonstrated the challenges of treatment (Figure 8.4b): the presence of branches at the proximal cap of the CTO and an unclear path of the vessel typical for a CTO in this location.

A Confianza Pro guidewire was engaged into the proximal cap of the lesion and then retracted into the CROSSER Catheter (Figure 8.4c). This is optimal positioning for advancement of the device. Excellent guide catheter support was critical, so that with the CROSSER device, advancement of the guide was firmly in place as a 'backstop'.

The CROSSER Catheter continued to advance with moderate resistance, and periodic contrast injections were taken to ascertain that the device was going in the appropriate direction (Figure 8.4d). At this point, the guidewire was advanced to attempt to reach the distal vessel.

A lateral view demonstrated that the CTO was successfully crossed (Figure 8.4e). One of the challenges in distal wire placement was entering (and having to avoid) the marginal branches.

The final result post-stenting is shown in Figure 8.4f. The mid to distal RCA segment, where the vessel courses under the heart, is one of the more complex segments to negotiate with a guidewire in the presence of a CTO. The CROSSER Catheter does not require manipulation; generally it seeks the lumen and, if not reaching it, is very difficult to advance forward.

CLINICAL STUDIES

Grube et al[8] reported on a total of 55 CTO lesions in 53 patients treated in Europe in two clinical phases:

1. A phase 1 feasibility study (30 CTOs), with a primary focus on device safety.
2. A phase 2 pivotal study (25 CTOs) using an improved version of the device, with a primary focus on effectiveness. This improved version of the device had a smaller tip (1.1 mm vs 1.3 mm) and a hydrophilic coating.

Among the 30 CTO lesions treated during the feasibility phase, the technical success rate was 47%, but device efficacy was only 40%. In two patients with RCA occlusions, the CROSSER Catheter crossed the CTO, but only made progress into a marginal branch distal to the occlusion; the distal segment of the vessel could not be wired. No major adverse events or complications relating to vibrational energy, either clinical or angiographic, occurred during the procedure or within a 30-day follow-up. In particular, there was no device-related perforation, thrombosis, abrupt closure, coronary artery spasm, side-branch loss, distal embolization, and no reflow, bradycardia, or hypotension. One patient experienced discomfort during the entire procedure, both with vibrational energy application and during contrast injection and balloon inflation. From the experience gathered

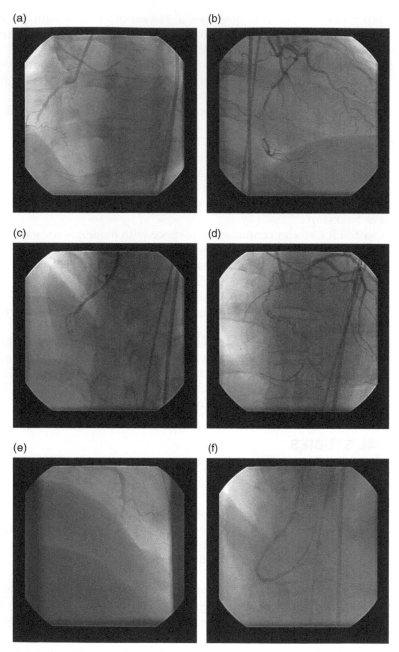

Figure 8.4   Repeated attempt to recanalize a right coronary artery. See text for step–by–step details.

during this phase, the limitations of the device were noted and addressed accordingly, resulting in the final version of the CROSSER Catheter that was used in the pivotal phase of the trial.

In the pivotal phase, using the improved version of the CROSSER Catheter, the primary endpoint of device efficacy was 76%, and the secondary endpoint of clinical success was also 76%. Overall, combining the results from both phases of the study, the device efficacy and clinical success were 56%. No death, Q-wave myocardial infarction (MI) or target vessel revascularization were observed; only two non-Q-wave MIs (NQMIs) were observed (3.8%). In particular, no coronary perforation or pericardial tamponade occurred. Procedure time was 83 ± 39 minutes, and average fluoroscopic time was 30 ± 18 minutes.

Melzi et al[9] reported on 28 patients with 30 chronic total occlusions. Most patients (92.8%) had TIMI (Thrombolysis in Myocardial Infarction) 0 flow. The age of the occlusion was clinically determined in seven (23%) and angiographically in 20 (67%) lesions. In three cases (10%), it was unknown. The median age of occlusion was 9 months and the mean occlusion length was 28 mm. The majority of the lesions had a blunt morphology. Overall technical success was obtained in 19 cases (63%) and angiographic success in 16 cases (53%): technical success using the CROSSER Catheter was 56% in lesions with a prior failed procedure and 67% in which the CROSSER Catheter was used in the same procedure following an initial unsuccessful guidewire attempt. Following successful reopening, all lesions were stented utilizing both bare metal and drug-eluting stents. Coronary guidewire perforation (type 1) occurred in one (3%) patient; despite this, the procedure was a clinical success. Only one patient (3%), who had an unsuccessful procedure, had a periprocedural MI. Clinical follow-up was available in all patients at 30 days. During the follow-up period, no additional major adverse cardiac events (MACE) occurred in any of the patients. The FACTOR coronary study was a recent prospective registry that was completed at 19 clinical centers in the USA. The study enrolled 125 patients with known chronic coronary occlusions, defined as occlusions documented to be in existence for >30 days All occlusions enrolled into the study were first probed with a wire to demonstrate resistance to conventional guidewire crossing. A more supportive, CTO specific guidewire was used for this attempt in 27% of the cases, whereas a soft or floppy wire was used in 29% of the attempts. The CROSSER Catheter was then delivered and activated at the CTO in an effort to cross the occlusion. An average of 156 seconds of activation time, as measured by the CROSSER electronics, was utilized for each crossing attempt. The CROSSER Catheter was able to facilitate guidewire crossing (defined as documentation of any conventional guidewire in the true distal lumen) in 61% of the cases. After crossing the occlusions and placing the guidewire in the true distal lumen of the vessel, normal PTCA/stenting was performed typically over that same guidewire. The study reported an 8.8% MACE rate and no clinical perforations. MACE was defined as NQMI (CPK >2×NL), Q-wave MI, death, repeat revascularization, and clinical perforation within 30 days. Overall, there were no device safety-related issues with the use of the CROSSER system. Results of this study were submitted to the US Food and Drug Administration (FDA) to support US marketing approval, and will be published in short order.

REFERENCES

1. Siegel RJ, DonMichael TA, Fishbein MC, et al. In vivo ultrasound arterial recanalization of atherosclerotic total occlusions. J Am Coll Cardiol 1990; 15:345–51.
2. Zocchi ML. Basic physics for ultrasound-assisted lipoplasty. Clin Plast Surg 1999; 26:209–20.
3. Rosenschein U, Bernstein JJ, DiSegni E, et al. Experimental ultrasonic angioplasty: disruption of atherosclerotic plaques and thrombi in vitro and arterial recanalization in vitro. J Am Coll Cardiol 1990; 15:711–17.
4. Fischell TA, Abbas MA, Grant GW, Siegal RJ. Ultrasonic energy. Effects on vascular function and integrity. Circulation 1991; 84:1783–95.
5. Siegel RJ, Cumberland DC, Myler RK, DonMichael TA. Percutaneous ultrasonic angioplasty: initial clinical experience. Lancet 1989; 2:772–4.
6. Cannon L, Siegel R, Greenberg J, et al. Recanalization of total coronary occlusions using the Sonicross low frequency ultrasound catheter. J Am Coll Cardiol 2000; 35:41A.
7. Cannon L, John J, LaLonde J. Therapeutic ultrasound for chronic total coronary occlusions. Echocardiography 2001; 18:219–23.
8. Grube E, Sütsch G, Lim VY, et al. High-frequency mechanical vibration to recanalize chronic total occlusions after failure to cross with conventional guidewires. J Invasive Cardiol 2006; 18(3):85–91.
9. Melzi G, Cosgrave J, Biondi-Zoccai GL, et al. A novel approach to chronic total occlusions: the CROSSER system. Catheter Cardiovasc Interv 2006; 68(1):29–35.

9

The role of fibrinolytic therapy in the management of chronic total occlusions

Amr E Abbas and William W O'Neill

As has been previously described, an atherosclerotic plaque is invariably present in chronic total occlusions (CTOs) and multiple layers of clot occur on top of episodes of plaque rupture/fissuring, accounting for the complete luminal occlusion.[1] The use of fibrinolytic therapy has been proposed as a mechanism to lyse the most recent clot component of CTO, allowing the passage of the guidewire and facilitating percutaneous coronary intervention (PCI).[2-7] This technique was initially described by Fergusson et al, with the use of streptokinase in the recanalization of a CTO of the right coronary artery.[2] This hypothesis has been subsequently tested in the occlusions of the peripheral circulation,[8] saphenous vein grafts,[9] and in the native coronary circulation.[3-7] Both fibrin-specific and fibrin-non-specific agents have been examined. This chapter highlights the use of intracoronary fibrinolytic therapy (ICL) in the recanalization and interventional management of CTO in the native coronary circulation, and also includes the treatment of chronically occluded aortocoronary saphenous vein grafts.

MECHANISM OF ACTION

Primary atherosclerotic disease develops over years to decades and the plaque is invariably present in de-novo occlusions as a minor or major part of the luminal obstruction. Occlusive or non-occlusive, single or multiple layers of clot of various ages then occur on top of episodes of plaque disruption/fissuring, and the most recent clot accounts for the complete occlusion. Microchannels may form within the occluded segment, and together with dilation of the vasa vasorum and clot lysis, may account for the presence of antegrade flow manifested as functional occlusion.[1] Successful PCI requires crossing through the clot and/or the microchannels. Fibrinolytic therapy may lyse the most recent clot component of the CTO and thus help 'soften' the plaque, allowing passage of the guidewire (Figure 9.1). Of interest, in patients with reocclusion following successful recanalization of CTO, depressed levels of endogenous tissue plasminogen activator levels (t-PA, indicating enhanced endogenous platelet reactivity) were found compared with patients without reocclusion.[10]

FIBRINOLYTIC AGENTS USED

Trials utilizing ICL in the management of CTO in the native coronary circulation are summarized in Table 9.1.

Non-fibrin-specific agents

Both streptokinase[2] and urokinase have been used.[3-6] Infusion of urokinase has been more extensively studied and its use has been described with either low dose (100 000 to 240 000 units) or high-dose (800 000 to 3.2 million units) preparations, and durations of 8–25 hours. The success rate appears independent of dose or duration of infusion. However, with higher doses, the incidence of bleeding complications is higher.

Fibrin-specific agents

Use of both tissue plasminogen activator (alteplase, t-PA) and tenecteplase (TNK) have been described,[7] with a weight-adjusted dose in the former and a standard dose in the latter. The duration of infusion has been limited in the studies to 8 hours. Despite the similar success rates for recanalization, the incidence of significant bleeding complications was markedly diminished compared with non-fibrin-specific agents. This may reflect the lower equivalent dose of the fibrin-specific agents used or may be related to shorter durations of infusions.

(a)   (b)

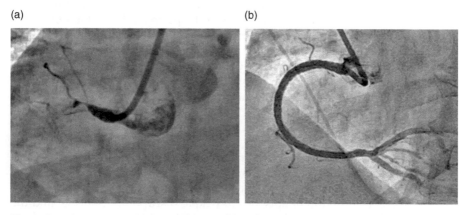

Figure 9.1   Angiograms demonstrating pre (a) and post (b) percutaneous coronary intervention (PCI) of the chronic total occlusion (CTO) of the right coronary artery (RCA). CTO angiographic characteristics include tapering, lack of bridging collaterals and side branch at the area of occlusion, proximal location, and no calcification. A total of three drug-eluting stents were implanted in an overlapping fashion from distal to proximal (3.5 × 33, 3.5 × 33, and 3.5 × 23) and a 4.0 non-compliant balloon was used for further expansion of the proximal stent.

Table 9.1 Comparison of non-fibrin-specific and fibrin-specific agents used for intracoronary lytic infusion prior to percutaneous coronary revascularization of chronic total occlusions (CTOs)

Agent used	Urokinase[3-6]	Fibrin–specific agent[7]
Dose	Bolus and infusion: 120 000 units bolus and 200 000 units/hour Low dose: 100 000 to 240 000 units High dose: 800 000 to 3.2 million units	Alteplase: 1–2.5 mg/hour Tenecteplase: 0.25 mg/hour
Duration of infusion	Bolus and infusion: 24 hours Low dose: 8–25 hours High dose: 8 hours	8 hours
Number of patients	Bolus and infusion: 20 Low dose: 25 patients High dose: 60 patients	85 patients Alteplase: 61 patients Tenecteplase: 24 patients
Success rate	Bolus and infusion: 85% Low dose: 52% High dose: 53%	54%
Serious bleeding complications	Bolus and infusion: ? Low dose: 8% High dose: 4–25%	3.5%
Population	CTO >3 months with previous unsuccessful attempt	CTO >3 months with previous unsuccessful attempt

TECHNIQUE

Patients undergo coronary angiography and a guide catheter with pre-manufactured side holes is placed in the target vessel. Over a guidewire, a 3 Fr intracoronary infusion catheter (ultrafuse catheter) is positioned at the face of the CTO. The total dose of the thrombolytic agent is divided between the infusion catheter and the guide catheter to prevent clot formation in the guide catheter (Figure 9.2). Intravenous heparin is administered during lytic infusion to achieve activated clotting time (ACT) levels between 200 and 250 seconds. The femoral sheath, guiding catheter, and ultrafuse catheter are securely sutured to the skin to ensure stability and covered with a sterile dressing. Patient immobility during the infusion is ensured to minimize bleeding and groin complications and adequate analgesia and sedation are administered to optimize patient comfort. Patients are observed in the coronary care unit during lytic infusion and are brought back to the laboratory. On their second visit, the sheath and catheters are exchanged for attempted recanalization using standard equipment.[7]

PREDICTORS OF SUCCESS

The success rate for recanalization of a CTO with a history of previous failed attempts is just over 50%.[2-7] The success rate seems to be independent of the lytic agent used or the duration of infusion. Figure 9.3 highlights the predictors of successful recanalization of CTOs with the use of ICL. Both these factors suggest that a favorable anatomy that would help deliver the lytic agent at the occlusion site

(a)   (b)

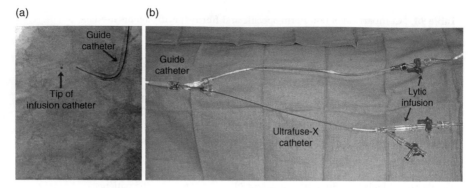

Figure 9.2   An angiogram (a) showing a guiding catheter situated in the right coronary artery. A guidewire is advanced in the vessel and a 3 Fr ultrafuse catheter is advanced to the site of occlusion. The guiding catheter and ultrafuse catheter (b) are sutured to the skin and covered in a sterile fashion.

by 'wedging' of the infusion catheter (tapering morphology) as well as the lack of dispersion of the lytic agent (absence of bridging collaterals) is essential for the success of this technique.[7]

SAFETY

As expected, groin hematomas and transfusion rates are higher with the use of ICL. The incidence of these complications has been reported to be as low as 3–4% in low-dose urokinase infusions and equivalent doses of fibrin-specific agents[6,7] and as high as 25% with the use of higher doses and longer infusions of urokinase.[6]

THROMBOLYTIC AGENTS FOR RECANALIZATION OF CHRONICALLY OCCLUDED SAPHENOUS VEIN GRAFTS

In a study of 46 patients with 47 totally occluded vein grafts, who received uroki-nase prior to recanalization attempts, and with a mean graft age of 7 years (range 1–13), the success rate was 79%. Patients received urokinase infusions delivered at a dose of 100 000 to 250 000 units/hour. The total dose of urokinase ranged from 0.7 to 9.8 million units over 7.5 to 77 hours (mean 31 hours). This study differs from those utilizing lytic infusions for CTOs of the native coronary circulation in that there were no prior attempts at recanalization. This may account in part for the higher success rate in this study.[9]

CONCLUSIONS

The use of ICL to facilitate recanalization of CTOs that have failed a previous attempt is successful in over 50% of cases in the coronary circulation. These studies have been conducted at single institutions and the success rate does not seem to be related to the type of thrombolytic agent or the duration of infusion. However, a lower incidence of complications is observed with the use of low-dose uroki-nase and fibrin-specific lytic agents compared with higher doses of urokinase.

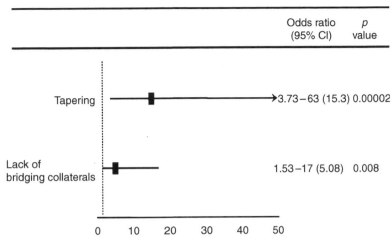

Figure 9.3 Multivariate predictors of successful recanalization of chronic total occlusions (CTOs) with intracoronary lytic (ICL) infusion in patients with previous failed attempts.

Delivery of an adequate dose of thrombolytic agent is essential and is enhanced by a tapering morphology of the occlusion and the lack of bridging collaterals. Thrombolytics should be considered as a valuable tool in the management of CTOs. A multicenter randomized trial is underway to test the benefit of lytic therapy prior to primary recanalization of de-novo coronary CTOs.

REFERENCES

1. Meier B. Chronic total occlusions. In: Topol EJ, ed. Textbook of Interventional Cardiology, 4th edn. Philadelphia: WB Saunders; 2003:303–16.
2. Ferguson DW, Kouba CR, Little MM, et al. Combined intracoronary streptokinase and percutaneous coronary angioplasty for reperfusion of chronic total coronary occlusion. J Am Coll Cardiol 1984; 4(4):820–14.
3. Cecena FA. Urokinase infusion after unsuccessful angioplasty in patients with chronic total occlusion of native coronary arteries. Cathet Cardiovasc Diagn 1993; 28(3):214–18.
4. Ajluni SC, Jones D, Zidar FJ, et al. Prolonged urokinase infusion for chronic total native coronary artery occlusions: clinical, angiographic, and treatment observations. Catheter Cardiovasc Diagn 1995; 34:106–10.
5. Kaplan BM, Zidar F, Jones D, et al. A prolonged intracoronary infusion of urokinase for chronic total occlusions: case reviews. J Invasive Cardiol 1995; 7 (Suppl E):21–25E.
6. Zidar FJ, Kaplan BM, O'Neill WW, et al. Prospective randomized trial of prolonged intracoronary urokinase infusion for chronic total occlusions in native arteries. J Am Coll Cardiol 1996; 27:1406–12.
7. Abbas AE, Brewington SD, Dixon SR, et al. Intracoronary fibrin-specific thrombolytic infusion facilitates percutaneous recanalization of chronic total occlusion. J Am Coll Cardiol 2005; 46(5):793–8.
8. Cragg AH, Smith TP, Corson JD, et al. Two urokinase dosing regimens in native arterial and graft occlusions: initial results of a prospective randomized clinical trial. Radiology 1991; 178:681–6.

9. Hartmann JR, McKeever LS, Stamato NJ, et al. Recanalization of chronically occluded aorto-coronary saphenous vein bypass grafts by extended infusion of urokinase: initial results and short-term clinical follow-up. J Am Coll Cardiol 1991; 18(6):1517–23.
10. Terres W, Lund GK, Hubner A, et al. Endogenous tissue plasminogen activator and platelet reactivity as risk factors for reocclusion after recanalization of chronic total coronary occlusions. Am Heart J 1995; 130(4):711–16.

10

Drug-eluting stents for chronic total occlusions: the European experience

Angela Hoye

Sirolimus-eluting stents for chronic total occlusions • **Paclitaxel-eluting stents for chronic total occlusions** • **Sirolimus-eluting stents vs paclitaxel-eluting stents** • **Summary**

Across Europe, interventional cardiology is expanding, with particularly rapid growth in the number of procedures in Eastern European countries.[1] In 2005, >1.3 million stents were implanted in Europe, of which drug-eluting stents (DESs) were used in approximately 45%. This proportion varies from country to country and unit to unit, with usage limited at present by the increased initial cost of these stents in comparison with bare metal stents (BMSs).

The first DES to receive Conformitè Europèenne (CE) mark approval for use in Europe was the sirolimus-eluting stent (SES) (Cypher, Cordis Johnson & Johnson), which was licensed from April 16, 2002. The efficacy of the stent relates to reducing restenosis through suppression of neointimal proliferation.[2,3] Preliminary randomized study evaluation of 238 patients demonstrated that, compared with its BMS counterpart, there was significantly lower late lumen loss at 6 months in the SES treated group (-0.01 ± 0.33 mm vs 0.8 ± 0.53 mm, $p < 0.001$).[3] In accordance with this angiographic efficacy and reduction in restenosis, the SES group had a significantly lower rate of major adverse cardiac events (MACE) at 1 year (5.8% vs 28.8%, $p < 0.001$). The second DES to receive CE mark approval in 2003 was the paclitaxel-eluting stent (PES) (Taxus, Boston Scientific Corp), which had similarly been evaluated in randomized studies. The preliminary TAXUS I trial demonstrated effective suppression of neointimal proliferation, with a late lumen loss of 0.36 ± 0.48 mm in the PES group vs 0.7 ± 0.48 mm in the BMS cohort.[4] However, patients treated in these landmark studies had relatively simple lesions, and those with complex disease such as chronic total occlusions (CTOs) were excluded.

Therapy for a CTO constitutes approximately 10% of angioplasty procedures, with this proportion remaining relatively stable over time since the mid-1990s.[5] Following successful recanalization, the long-term outcome of CTO therapy is hampered by a comparatively increased rate of adverse events,[6] with a relatively high rate of restenosis and reocclusion. In the 1990s, several randomized studies demonstrated that results following stent implantation were superior compared with treatment with balloon-only angioplasty.[7-11] However, restenosis rates remained in the order of 32–55%, with reocclusion occurring in up to 12%. As soon as DES received CE mark approval, several centers in Europe evaluated their efficacy in the treatment of complex lesions such as CTOs. An overview of the clinical and angiographic results from several of these recent European studies is summarized in Table 10.1.

SIROLIMUS-ELUTING STENTS FOR CHRONIC TOTAL OCCLUSIONS

The RESEARCH Registry

The first data demonstrating effectiveness of the SES for CTOs came from registry data. Following CE mark approval, all consecutive patients treated at the Thoraxcenter in Rotterdam received the SES irrespective of patient or lesion characteristics (the RESEARCH Registry). During the first 6 months, 56 consecutive patients received SES implantation following successful recanalization of a CTO (defined as >1 months' duration).[12] The cohort was compared with the group of patients treated for CTO with BMS implantation during the 6-month period immediately prior to the introduction of SES ($n = 28$). The groups were evaluated for the occurrence of MACE defined, as death, acute myocardial infarction (AMI), or target vessel revascularization (TVR). There were no significant differences between the groups in terms of the baseline patient characteristics. At 12 months, there was a significantly higher rate of survival-free of MACE in the SES group (96.4% vs 82.1% in the BMS group, $p < 0.05$) (Figure 10.1). At 6 months, the SES group ($n = 33$) underwent follow-up angiography. The results demonstrated highly effective suppression of neointimal proliferation, with an overall binary restenosis rate of 9% and in-stent late loss of 0.13 ± 0.46 mm (see Table 10.1). There was a single reocclusion (3%).

The Milan experience

Following this preliminary evidence, further registry data were published from Milan.[13] In a similar fashion to Rotterdam, 122 patients treated with SES between April 2002 and April 2004 were compared with all consecutive patients ($n = 259$) treated with BMS implantation for a CTO in the 24 months prior to the introduction of the SES. Patients were included if the occlusion was estimated to be at least 3 months in duration. Baseline patient characteristics were similar, except that those treated during the latter period were significantly more likely to be smokers and have hypercholesterolemia. Notably, those treated with DESs had longer lesions, and were treated with significantly longer length of stent(s), which is potentially unfavorable in terms of restenosis – in the era of the BMS, the longer-stented segment is known to be a predictor of restenosis.[14] The large ratio of stent length to lesion length in the SES group can be attributed to the desire of the operator to completely cover the lesion. Despite this, follow-up

Table 10.1   Overview of recent European studies evaluating drug-eluting stent implantation for chronic total occlusions

Parameter	RESEARCH Registry SES[12]	Milan Registry			PRISON II			Werner et al		
		BMS[13]	SES[13]	p value	BMS[17]	SES[17]	p value	BMS[19]	PES[19]	p value
Mean number of stents/lesion	2.0	1.2	1.4	0.002	1.4	1.4	ns	1.7	1.7	0.91
Mean diameter of stent/final balloon (mm)	2.75 ± 0.26	3.19 ± 0.48	2.97 ± 0.42	<0.001	3.32 ± 0.39	3.18 ± 0.32	n/a	3.04 ± 0.44	2.95 ± 0.38	0.26
Mean total length of stent(s) used (mm)	45 ± 25	22 ± 9	42 ± 20	<0.001	29 ± 14	32 ± 15	n/a	36 ± 21	40 ± 19	0.33
Clinical outcomes										
Number of patients	56	259	122		100	100		48	48	
Follow-up duration (months)	12	6	6		6	6		12	12	
Death (%)	0	1	3	0.61	0	0	–	4	2	ns
AMI (%)	2	8	8	0.97	3	2	ns	2	4	ns
TLR (%)	4	26	7	<0.001	19	4	0.001	44	6	<0.001
MACE (%)	4	35	16	<0.001	20	4	<0.001	48	13	<0.001
30-day stent thrombosis (%)	2	0.4	0	0.70	0	1	ns	0	0	–
Angiographic outcomes										
Number of patients	33	228	119		94	94		48	47	
Ref. vessel diameter (mm)	2.58 ± 0.55	2.78 ± 0.67	2.89 ± 0.46	0.12	3.26 ± 0.52	3.38 ± 0.55	ns	2.65 ± 0.65	2.57 ± 0.47	0.51
Post-procedure MLD (mm)	2.04 ± 0.45	2.69 ± 0.53	2.67 ± 0.49	0.77	2.55 ± 0.43	2.53 ± 0.56	ns	2.16 ± 0.60	2.26 ± 0.36	0.32
Follow-up MLD (mm)	1.91 ± 0.68	1.63 ± 0.98	2.39 ± 0.88	<0.001	1.47 ± 0.83	2.48 ± 0.80	<0.0001	1.00 ± 0.73	2.05 ± 0.59	<0.001
Post-procedure DS (%)	13	12	13	0.12	15	19	0.001	15	11	0.17
Follow-up DS (%)	22	44	18	<0.001	49	22	<0.0001	59	20	<0.001
Late lumen loss (mm)	0.13 ± 0.46	1.04 ± 0.87	0.28 ± 0.56	<0.001	1.09 ± 0.91	0.05 ± 0.81	<0.0001	1.21 ± 0.70	0.19 ± 0.62	<0.001
Binary restenosis rate (%)	9	33	9	<0.001	36	7	<0.001	51	8	<0.001
Reocclusion (%)	3	7	3	0.17	13	4	<0.04	23	2	0.003

AMI, acute myocardial infarction; DS, diameter of stenosis; MACE, major adverse cardiac events; MLD, minimal lumen diameter; n/a, not available, ns, not significant; TLR, target lesion revascularization.

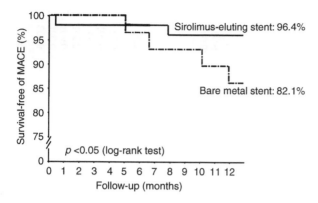

Figure 10.1 Cumulative survival-free of major adverse cardiac events (MACE) for patients with a chronic total occlusion treated with implantation of sirolimus-eluting and bare metal stents. (Reproduced from Hoye et al,[12] with permission.)

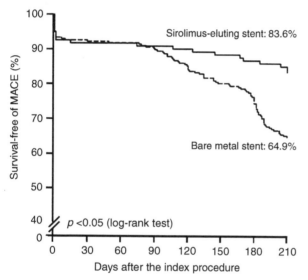

Figure 10.2 Cumulative survival-free of major adverse cardiac events (MACE) for patients with a chronic total occlusion treated with implantation of sirolimus-eluting and bare metal stents. (Reproduced from Ge et al,[13] with permission.)

angiography at 6 months demonstrated efficacy of the SES, with a significantly smaller late lumen loss and a significantly lower restenosis rate (see Table 10.1).

At 6 months the clinical results demonstrated a rate of survival-free of MACE of 83.6% in the SES group vs 64.9% in the BMS group ($p < 0.001$) – Figure 10.2. There were no differences between the groups in the occurrence of cardiac death or AMI, with the difference in MACE therefore relating to significantly fewer TLRs in the SES group (7% vs 26%, $p < 0.001$).

The e-Cypher Registry

With the widespread introduction of the SES, the e-Cypher post-marketing surveillance registry was introduced to evaluate the clinical outcomes of patients treated in daily practice. Patients were included from 281 centers in 41 countries, with an independent committee to adjudicate all events. Of 15 172 patients, 350 patients (2.3%) were treated only for at least one CTO lesion (defined as a duration >3 months).[15] The mean number of stents was 1.4. Compared with the

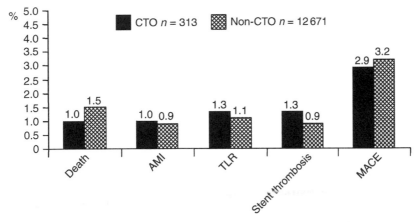

Figure 10.3 Incidence of adverse cardiac events in the e-Cypher Registry for patients treated for a chronic total occlusion as compared with those treated for other lesion subtypes. AMI, acute myocardial infarction; CTO, chronic total occlusion; TLR, target lesion revascularization; MACE, major adverse cardiac events.

patients treated for non-CTO lesions (n = 14 735), those treated for CTO lesions had a significantly smaller mean reference diameter (2.83 ± 0.31 mm vs 2.87 ± 0.36 mm, $p < 0.05$), and a significantly longer mean lesion length (25.6 ± 12.0 mm vs 17.0 ± 8.6 mm, $p < 0.05$). Despite this, the clinical outcomes at 6 months were similar in both groups (Figure 10.3). At 12 months, the survival-free of MACE in the CTO group was 93.5%, with target lesion revascularization undertaken in just 2.9%.

The SICTO study

The SICTO (CYPHER Sirolimus-eluting stent in Chronic Total Occlusion) study[16] was a multicenter study with a detailed assessment of 25 patients to include both angiographic and intravascular ultrasound (IVUS) follow-up, with a primary endpoint of in-stent late loss at 6 months. The reference vessel diameter was 2.6 ± 0.5 mm, and mean stent length 28 ± 11 mm. At 6 months, the primary endpoint of mean in-stent late loss was −0.03 mm ± 0.28 mm with a binary restenosis rate of 0%. Paired data from IVUS evaluations similarly showed efficacy in suppression of neointimal proliferation (Table 10.2). At 12 months, no patient died or suffered a myocardial infarction. A single patient underwent target lesion revascularization (TLR) (4%).

The PRISON II study

A pivotal study in the evaluation of the SES has been the PRISON II study carried out in two centers in Amsterdam.[17] Following successful CTO recanalization, 200 patients were randomized to receive either the SES or the bare metal (Bx VELOCITY) stent. The groups were well matched in terms of baseline patient characteristics and angiographic characteristics such as mean occlusion length. The primary endpoint was binary restenosis at 6 months, with angiographic assessment carried out at an independent core laboratory. All patients were treated with aspirin

Table 10.2 Results of intravascular ultrasound evaluation from the SICTO study of patients treated with sirolimus-eluting stent implantation for a chronic total occlusion

	Post-procedure	6-month follow-up
Mean stent area (mm²)	8.6 ± 1.8	8.7 ± 1.7
Mean lumen area (mm²)	8.6 ± 1.8	8.3 ± 1.9
Minimal lumen area (mm²)	6.7 ± 1.7	6.4 ± 2.2
Percent stent plaque volume (mm³)	–	13.1 ± 18.3

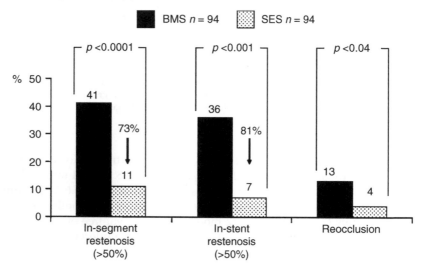

Figure 10.4 Reduction in restenosis and reocclusion rates following sirolimus-eluting stent implantation compared with bare metal stent implantation in the randomized PRISON II study of chronic total occlusions. BMS, bare metal stent; SES, sirolimus-eluting stent.

100 mg/day, together with clopidogrel 75 mg/day for at least 6 months. There was a statistically significant difference between the two groups in favor of the SES (Figure 10.4), with a 73% relative risk reduction in in-segment restenosis (11% vs 41%, $p < 0.0001$). The results of the 6-month quantitative coronary angiography evaluation are presented in Table 10.1. In terms of the clinical outcomes, there were significantly fewer adverse events in the SES group related to a lower rate of TLR (4% vs 19%, $p = 0.001$)(Figure 10.5). Such strong evidence from a well-conducted randomized study has provided clear evidence of efficacy of the SES in this complex lesion subgroup, and follow-up is planned to evaluate the long-term outcomes at 24 months.

The CORACTO study

CTO lesions were also the target lesion of the CORACTO study,[18] which evaluated the sirolimus-coated CURA stent in 95 patients with a CTO of >3 months' duration. The stent has a biodegradeable polymer coating 3.5 μm thick, with sirolimus at a dose of 170 ± 20 μg/cm². Patients were randomized to treatment

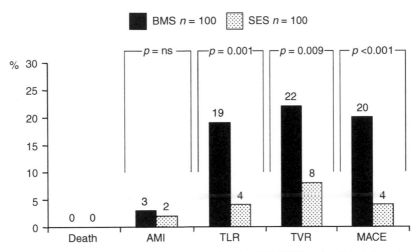

Figure 10.5   Clinical outcomes of patients treated in the PRISON II study of chronic total occlusions. Comparison patients treated with sirolimus-eluting and bare metal stent implantation. AMI, acute myocardial infarction; TLR, target lesion revascularization; TVR, target vessel revascularization; MACE, major adverse cardiac events.

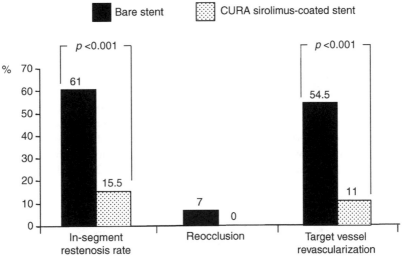

Figure 10.6   Results of the randomized CORACTO study comparing the CURA sirolimus-coated stent with bare metal stent implantation in the treatment of chronic total occlusions.

with either the CURA stent or BMS implantation. The primary endpoint was late loss and restenosis at 6 months, with angiographic analysis undertaken at a core laboratory. Stents were 17 mm long, and the mean total stent length used was 47.6 mm (2.8 stents/patient). Follow-up angiography demonstrated significant differences between the two groups in favor of the CURA stent. The mean late loss was 1.46 mm in those treated with the bare stent vs 0.41 mm in the CURA stent group ($p < 0.001$). The suppression of neointimal proliferation was associated with less restenosis, reocclusion, and need for TVR (Figure 10.6). Importantly, no patient died or suffered a stent thrombosis or myocardial infarction.

PACLITAXEL-ELUTING STENTS FOR CHRONIC TOTAL OCCLUSIONS

The PES was introduced into European practice in early 2003. Werner et al evaluated the efficacy of this stent in 48 consecutive patients treated for a CTO as compared with a matched group of 48 patients previously treated with BMS.[19] Patients were matched on the basis of a history of diabetes mellitus, prior MI, diameter and number of stents implanted, lesion location, and left ventricular function, and were drawn from a total of 148 patients treated in the preceding 4 years.

The clinical outcomes are presented in Table 10.1. All three deaths occurred in patients with severe impairment of left ventricle (LV) function. The PES-treated group had significantly fewer adverse events relating to the reduced need for repeat revascularization (Figure 10.7). The authors noted that diabetic patients treated with BMS had almost double the rate of target vessel failure compared with non-diabetic patients (64% vs 35%). However, this difference was not apparent in the diabetic population treated with PES (6% vs 9%). The advantage of the PES over BMS was significant both in diabetic and non-diabetic patients. Angiographic follow-up demonstrated the efficacy of the PES with a significantly smaller late lumen loss in the PES-treated group, and significantly less restenosis (8% vs 51%) and reocclusion (2% vs 23%) (see Table 10.1).

SIROLIMUS-ELUTING STENTS VS PACLITAXEL-ELUTING STENTS

The clinical outcomes of both the SESs and PESs for the treatment of CTOs were further analyzed in the registry data from Rotterdam, whereby, from April 2002, all patients were treated with DESs. All consecutive patients treated for a CTO of >3 months' duration were included in the study.[20] A cohort of 76 patients were treated with the SES; subsequently, in the first quarter of 2003, all patients were

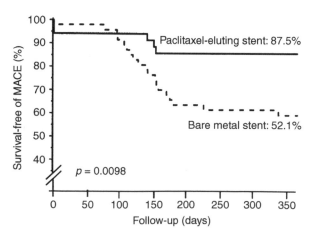

Figure 10.7 Cumulative survival-free of major adverse cardiac events (MACE) for patients with a chronic total occlusion treated with implantation of paclitaxel-eluting and bare metal stents. (Reprinted from Jam Coll Cardiol, Vol 44, Werner GS, Knack A, Schwarz G, et al. Prevention of lesion recurrence in chronic total coronary occlusions by paclitaxel-eluting stents. Pages 2301–6. 2004. With Permission from the American College of Cardiology foundation.)[19]

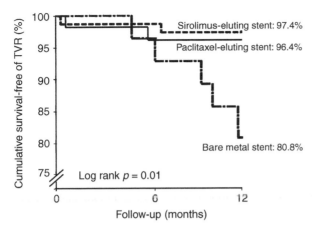

Figure 10.8 Cumulative survival-free of target vessel revascularization (TVR) following chronic total occlusion treatment with sirolimus-eluting, paclitaxel-eluting, or bare metal stent implantation. (Reproduced from Hoye et al,[20] with permission.)

treated with the PES, including 57 treated for a CTO. Both groups of DES patients were compared with a similar group of patients treated with BMS ($n = 26$) in the preceding 6-month period prior to the introduction of the SES. Patients treated in the DES era were treated with a greater number of stents (2.2 ± 1.2 for SES, 2.6 ± 1.3 for PES, 1.8 ± 0.8 for BMS, $p = 0.03$), with a longer mean total length of stents (48.8 ± 27.4 mm for SES, 58.0 ± 32.8 mm for PES, 41.5 ± 23.3 mm for BMS, $p = 0.04$), and a smaller nominal stent diameter (2.8 ± 0.3 mm for SES, 2.8 ± 0.4 mm for PES, 3.0 ± 0.6 mm for BMS, $p < 0.001$). Despite these differences, which might potentially favor results in the BMS group, at 400 days, both DES groups had a significantly higher rate of survival-free of TVR compared with those treated with BMS (Figure 10.8).

De Lezo et al performed a randomized study of 144 patients with CTOs to treatment with either the SES or PES. The clinical and angiographic follow-up results of 65 of these patients (68 lesions) have been recently presented.[21] There were no significant differences in the baseline angiographic and procedural characteristics. Angiographic follow-up at 8 months demonstrated a restenosis rate of 6% for SES vs 17% for PES ($p = $ ns); however, the PES group were found to have a significantly higher late loss (0.49 ± 0.54 mm vs 0.23 ± 0.3 mm, $p < 0.05$), and neointimal area on IVUS (0.63 ± 0.5 mm^3 versus 1.3 ± 1.59 mm^3, $p < 0.05$). This difference was not associated with a disparity in the clinical outcomes; at 15 months there was a single death (in the PES group), no AMI (in either group), and a TLR rate of 3% (SES) vs 6% (PES), $p = $ ns.

SUMMARY

Both the SES and PES have shown safety and efficacy in improving outcomes in patients treated for a CTO. This improvement in outcomes relates to the development of significantly less restenosis, less re-occlusion and the need for significantly fewer repeat revascularizations. Most data relates to efficacy demonstrated in registry data, comparing these stents with patients treated historically with BMS prior to the introduction of the DES. There are, however, prospective randomized data of the SES in the PRISON II study. Figure 10.9 depicts significantly less need for repeat revascularization in patients treated in European Studies of

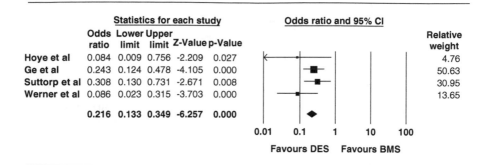

Figure 10.9   Need for target vessel revascularization in patients treated in European studies comparing drug-eluting stent (DES) versus bone metal stent (BMS) implantation for the treatment of chronic total occlusions. Odds ratio and 95% confidence invervals (CI) are shown.

DES implantation compared with bare metal stents. There are several other DES that have recently also been given CE mark approval; data regarding their use in more complex lesions such as CTOs are pending.

REFERENCES

1. Cook S, Togni M, Walpoth N, et al. Percutaneous coronary interventions in Europe 1992–2003. Eurointervention 2006; 1:374–9.
2. Sousa JE, Costa MA, Abizaid AC, et al. Sustained suppression of neointimal proliferation by sirolimus-eluting stents: one-year angiographic and intravascular ultrasound follow-up. Circulation 2001; 104:2007–11.
3. Morice MC, Serruys PW, Sousa JE, et al. A randomized comparison of a sirolimus-eluting stent with a standard stent for coronary revascularization. N Engl J Med 2002; 346:1773–80.
4. Grube E, Silber S, Hauptmann KE, et al. TAXUS I: six- and twelve-month results from a randomized, double-blind trial on a slow-release paclitaxel-eluting stent for de novo coronary lesions. Circulation 2003; 107:38–42.
5. Hoye A, van Domburg RT, Sonnenschein K, et al. Percutaneous coronary intervention for chronic total occlusions: the Thoraxcenter experience 1992–2002. Eur Heart J 2005; 26:2630–6.
6. Wilensky RL, Selzer F, Johnston J, et al. Relation of percutaneous coronary intervention of complex lesions to clinical outcomes (from the NHLBI Dynamic Registry). Am J Cardiol 2002; 90:216–21.
7. Rubartelli P, Niccoli L, Verna E, et al. Stent implantation versus balloon angioplasty in chronic coronary occlusions: results from the GISSOC trial. Gruppo Italiano di Studio sullo Stent nelle Occlusioni Coronariche. J Am Coll Cardiol 1998; 32:90–6.
8. Sirnes PA, Golf S, Myreng Y, et al. Stenting in Chronic Coronary Occlusion (SICCO): a randomized, controlled trial of adding stent implantation after successful angioplasty. J Am Coll Cardiol 1996; 28:1444–51.
9. Hoher M, Wohrle J, Grebe OC, et al. A randomized trial of elective stenting after balloon recanalization of chronic total occlusions. J Am Coll Cardiol 1999; 34:722–9.
10. Lotan C, Rozenman Y, Hendler A, et al. Stents in total occlusion for restenosis prevention. The multicentre randomized STOP study. The Israeli Working Group for Interventional Cardiology. Eur Heart J 2000; 21:1960–6.
11. Buller CE, Dzavik V, Carere RG, et al. Primary stenting versus balloon angioplasty in occluded coronary arteries: the Total Occlusion Study of Canada (TOSCA). Circulation 1999; 100:236–42.
12. Hoye A, Tanabe K, Lemos, PA et al. Significant reduction in restenosis after the use of sirolimus-eluting stents in the treatment of chronic total occlusions. J Am Coll Cardiol 2004; 43:1954–8.

13. Ge L, Iakovou I, Cosgrave J, et al. Immediate and mid-term outcomes of sirolimus-eluting stent implantation for chronic total occlusions. Eur Heart J 2005; 26:1056–62.
14. Kobayashi Y, De Gregorio J, Kobayashi N, et al. Stented segment length as an independent predictor of restenosis. J Am Coll Cardiol 1999; 34:651–9.
15. Lotan C, Gershlick AH, Guagliumi G, et al. Treatment of chronic total occlusion with the Sirolimus-eluting stent: 12-month results from the e-CYPHER Registry. Presented at American College of Cardiology (ACC), Scientific Session, Orlando; 2005.
16. Lotan C. The SICTO Study: Sirolimus-eluting stent in Chronic Total Occlusion. Presented at Transcatheter Cardiovascular Therapeutics (TCT) meeting, Washington; 2004.
17. Suttorp MJ, Laarman GJ. Primary stenting of occluded native coronary arteries, the PRISON II study. Presented at Transcatheter Cardiovascular Therapeutics (TCT) meeting, Washington; 2005.
18. Reifart N. Constant Stent (Neich) with Rapamycine in chronic total occlusions, the CORACTO trial. Presented at Transcatheter Cardiovascular Therapeutics (TCT) meeting, Washington; 2005.
19. Werner GS, Krack A, Schwarz G, et al. Prevention of lesion recurrence in chronic total coronary occlusions by paclitaxel-eluting stents. J Am Coll Cardiol 2004; 44:2301–6.
20. Hoye A, Ong ATL, Aoki J, et al. Drug-eluting stent implantation for chronic total occlusions: comparison between the sirolimus- and paclitaxel-eluting stent. Eurointervention 2005; 1:193–7.
21. de Lezo JS, Medina A, Pan M, et al. Drug-eluting stents for the treatment of chronic total occlusions. A randomized comparison of rapamycin- versus paclitaxel-eluting stents. Presented at American Heart Association (AHA) Scientific Sessions, Dallas; 2005.
22. Rahel BM, Suttorp MJ, Laarman GJ, et al. Primary stenting of occluded native coronary arteries: final results of the Primary Stenting of Occluded Native Coronary Arteries (PRISON) study. Am Heart J 2004; 147:e22.

11

Drug-eluting stents for chronic total occlusions: the North American and Asian experience

David E Kandzari

Rationale for DES implantation in CTO lesions • Contemporary DES trials in CTO revascularization • Comparative DES trials in CTO revascularization • Summary

Although a chronic total occlusion (CTO) is identified in approximately one-third up to one-half of diagnostic cardiac catheterizations, still an attempted revascularization accounts for generally less than 10% of all percutaneous coronary interventions (PCIs).[1,2] Such a disparity between their frequency and treatment not only underscores the technical and procedural frustrations associated with these complex lesions but also the clinical uncertainties regarding the clinical benefits of CTO revascularization and the ongoing inadequacies of conventional PCI methods for sustaining restenosis-free patency following initial success. The aims of this chapter therefore are to review the rationale for treatment with drug-eluting stents (DESs) in CTO revascularization; summarize recent DES clinical trial results, primarily from North America; and describe future directions for investigation.

RATIONALE FOR DES IMPLANTATION IN CTO LESIONS

In spite of the current widespread use of the DES beyond approved patient and lesion indications, until recently, few investigations have been performed to support the clinical benefit of the DES in CTO revascularization. In contrast, several previous trials comparing balloon angioplasty with bare metal stent placement have been completed[3-10] (Table 11.1). Although these trials have varied considerably regarding enrollment criteria, antithrombotic regimen, and trial design, their results are remarkably concordant, demonstrating statistically significant reductions in angiographic restenosis, reocclusion, and the need for repeat intervention associated with coronary stenting. However, these studies have also raised attention to the limitations unique to coronary occlusions, demonstrating that while stenting reduced angiographic and clinical adverse events compared with

Table 11.1 Randomized clinical trials of angioplasty vs stenting for chronic total coronary occlusions

Trial	n	Reocclusion			Restenosis			Target vessel revascularization		
		PTCA	Stent	p value	PTCA	Stent	p value	PTCA	Stent	p value
Stenting in Chronic Coronary Occlusion (SICCO)[4]	114	26%	16%	0.058	74%	32%	<0.001	42%	22%	0.025
Gruppo Italiano di Studi sulla Stent nelle Occlusioni Coronariche (GISSOC)[6]	110	34%	8%	0.004	68%	32%	0.0008	22%	5%	0.04
Mori et al[7]	96	11%	7%	0.04	57%	28%	0.005	49%	28%	<0.05
Stent vs Percutaneous Angioplasty in Chronic Total Occlusion (SPACTO)[5]	85	24%	3%	0.01	64%	32%	0.01	40%	25%	NS
Total Occlusion Study of Canada (TOSCA)[3]	410	20%	11%	0.02	70%	55%	<0.01	15%	8%	0.03
Stents in Total Occlusion for Restenosis Prevention (STOP)[8]	96	17%	8%	NS	71%	42%	0.032	42%	25%	NS
Stent or Angioplasty After Recanalization of Chronic Coronary Occlusions (SARECCO)[10]	110	14%	2%	0.05	62%	26%	0.01	55%	24%	0.05
Primary Stenting of Occluded Native Coronary Arteries (PRISON)[9]	200	7%	8%	0.99	33%	22%	0.14	29%	13%	<0.0001

PTCA, percutaneous transluminal coronary angioplasty; NS, not significant.

balloon angioplasty, intermediate and long-term outcomes following successful stent placement were still inferior to those observed among patients treated for non-occlusive lesions. In the Total Occlusion Study of Canada-1 (TOSCA-1) trial, for example, 6-month rates of restenosis and reocclusion in complex lesions exceeded 50% and 10%, respectively.[3] At 3-year follow-up in this trial, the occurrence of reocclusion was associated with a trend toward higher mortality and a significant increase in the need for repeat revascularization.[11]

While the lesion complexity of CTOs cannot be altered, however, the potential for new stent designs to improve rates of restenosis and reocclusion is considerable. The observations that (1) advances in the CTO technical and procedural success have been disproportionate to the increasing number of PCI procedures that involve non-acute occlusions, and (2) outcomes with conventional, bare metal stenting in CTOs are persistently inferior to stenting in non-occlusive lesions mandate the need for systematic evaluation of DES in CTO revascularization. In randomized clinical trials and in large cohort studies, failure to achieve or sustain patency after CTO recanalization has been associated with impairment in regional and global left ventricular systolic function, recurrent angina and target vessel revascularization, and a greater need for late bypass surgery.[12] Considering the potential for DES to inhibit neointimal proliferation, the implications of improving long-term restenosis-free patency in coronary occlusions are therefore significant.

CONTEMPORARY DES TRIALS IN CTO REVASCULARIZATION

At present only one randomized trial comparing DES with bare metal stents has been performed. In the Primary Stenting of Occluded Native Coronary Arteries (PRISON) II trial, 200 TCO patients were randomized in a single-blinded fashion at two centers in the Netherlands to treatment with either sirolimus-eluting stents (SESs; Cypher, Cordis Corporation, Miami Lakes, FL) or the bare metal BX VELOCITY stent (Cordis Corporation).[13] Overall, diabetes mellitus was present in 13% of patients, the age of total occlusions was <3 months in 55% of patients, and the average lesion and stent lengths were approximately 16 mm and 30 mm, respectively. At 6 months, treatment with SES was associated with statistically significant reductions in both in-stent (36% vs 7%, p <0.0001) and in-segment (41% vs 11%, p <0.001) angiographic restenosis (Figure 11.1). Reocclusion was also significantly reduced with SES (13% vs 4%, p <0.04), despite treatment in both groups with aspirin and clopidogrel for a minimum duration of 6 months. In parallel with the improvement in angiographic measures, similar benefit was observed in clinical outcome; specifically, target lesion revascularization at 6 months occurred in 19% and 4% of bare metal and SES-treated patients, respectively (p = 0.001 for comparison; Figure 11.2).

DES CTO registries

Several recent modest-sized observational studies examining clinical outcomes among patients treated with DES following successful CTO recanalization have supported the notion that, unlike bare metal stents, DES may achieve similar

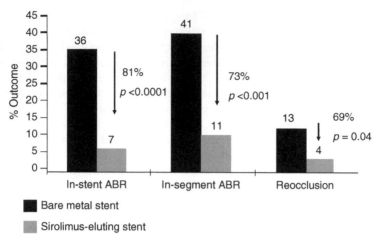

Figure 11.1 Six-month angiographic results from the PRISON II trial. ABR, angiographic binary restenosis.

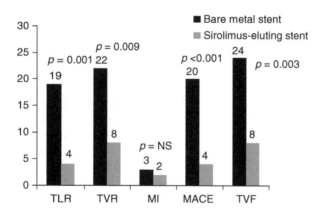

Figure 11.2 Six-month clinical outcomes from the PRISON II trial. TLR, target lesion revascularization; TVR, target vessel revascularization; MI, myocardial infarction; MACE, major adverse cardiac events; TVF, target vessel failure.

reductions in the need for repeat target vessel revascularization, as observed in non-occlusive lesions (Table 11.2). In the Sirolimus-eluting stent in Chronic Total Occlusion (SICTO) Study, treatment with SES in 25 patients undergoing successful total occlusion recanalization was associated with a 6-month target lesion revascularization rate of 8.0% (two patients) and no occurrence of stent thrombosis.[14] Angiographic in-stent late loss at 6 months was −0.1 ± 0.3 mm, a comparable angiographic result with SES in less-complex lesion morphologies.

In the RESEARCH Registry, among 56 patients treated with SES following CTO revascularization, the 1-year occurrence of repeat target vessel revascularization was 3.6%, compared with 17.9% among an historical control group of patients receiving bare metal stents.[15] Similarly, the 6-month rate of target lesion revascularization was only 1.4% for 360 patients with CTOs who were included in the prospective e-Cypher Registry.[16]

Table 11.2 Clinical trials evaluating drug-eluting stents in total coronary occlusions

Trial	*n*	Angiographic restenosis (%)	Target vessel revascularization (%)	Major adverse cardiac events (%)	Target vessel revascularization (%)	Major adverse cardiac events (%)
			6 months		1 year	
SICTO[14]	25	0	8.0	0	–	–
e-Cypher Registry[16]	360	–	1.4[a]	3.1	–	–
RESEARCH Registry[15]	56	9.1	3.6	3.6	–	–
Werner et al[20]	48	8.3	–	–	6.3	12.5
Nakamura et al[18]	60	2.0	3.0	–	3.0	–
Ge et al[19]	122	9.2	9.0	16.4	–	1.7
WISDOM Registry[21]	65	–	–	–	6.7	–
TRUE Registry[b22]	183	17.0	16.9	17.1	–	–

[a]Denotes target lesion revascularization.
[b]7-month clinical and angiographic outcomes reported.

Experience in Asia

Among 180 patients undergoing SES implantation for CTO revascularization in Asia, the 6-month occurrences of angiographic binary restenosis and target vessel revascularization were 1.5% and 2.3%, respectively.[17] As part of a multicenter Asian registry evaluating DES, clinical and angiographic outcomes among 60 patients who underwent SES implantation during CTO revascularization were compared with a matched control of 120 CTO patients treated with bare metal stents.[18] At 6-month clinical and angiographic follow-up, treatment with SES was associated with significant reductions in in-stent late loss, restenosis, and reocclusion. Target lesion revascularization was significantly lower at 6 months (23.0% vs 2.0%, $p = 0.001$), and the left ventricular ejection fraction also significantly improved among the SES patients (51.8% baseline vs 57.0% at 6 months, $p < 0.01$), this latter finding implying that maintenance of vessel patency with DES may be an important predictor of the improvement in left ventricular function. At 1 year, treatment with SES was associated with sustained reductions in hierarchical major adverse events (3.0% vs 42.0%, $p = 0.001$) and target lesion revascularization (43.0% vs 3.0%, $p = 0.001$).

In a retrospective study of 122 patients with chronic total occlusions treated with SES, clinical and angiographic outcomes were compared with an historical control of 259 patients treated with bare metal stents.[19] At 6 months, overall major adverse cardiac events were significantly lower among SES-treated patients (16.4% vs 35.1%, $p < 0.001$), principally due to a significantly lower rate of repeat target lesion revascularization (7.4% vs 26.3%, $p < 0.001$). Restenosis was identified in 9.2% of patients in the SES group and 33.3% in the bare metal stent group ($p < 0.001$). By multivariate analysis, significant predictors of 6-month major adverse events were the use of bare metal stents (hazard ratio [HR] 2.97; 95% confidence interval [CI] 1.80–4.89), lesion length (HR 2.02; 95% CI 1.37–2.99), and reference vessel diameter >2.8 mm (HR 0.62; 95% CI 0.42–0.92).

Paclitaxel-eluting stent for CTO

In addition to the study by Werner et al[20] that is discussed elsewhere, two additional registries studied paclitaxel-eluting stents (PESs) in CTO. Among 65 patients with CTOs in the international WISDOM Registry, treatment with the PES resulted in freedom from major adverse cardiac events and repeat intervention at 1 year in 93.3% and 98.3% of patients, respectively.[21] In the European TRUE Registry, among 183 patients with total occlusions who were treated with PES, 7-month rates of restenosis and target vessel revascularization were 17.0% and 16.9%, respectively.[22] Notably, the mean ($\pm$ standard deviation) number of stents per patient (2.2 $\pm$ 1.2) and total stent length (58 $\pm$ 33 mm) in this study were considerably greater than previous DES trials involving treatment of less-complex lesion subsets.

COMPARATIVE DES TRIALS IN CTO REVASCULARIZATION

Whether safety, clinical efficacy, and angiographic outcomes are similar between differing DESs have only been recently examined.[23-29] Despite more predictable variance in measures of neointimal hyperplasia by angiography and intravascular

Table 11.3 Comparative drug-eluting stent trials in total coronary occlusions

Trial	n	Angiographic restenosis (%)		Target vessel revascularization (%)		Major adverse cardiac events (%)	
		SES	PES	SES	PES	SES	PES
RESEARCH/ T-SEARCH Registry[30a]	76 SES, 57 PES	–	–	2.6	3.6	–	–
Nalamura et al, Asian Registry[31a]	396 SES, 526 PES	4.0	6.7	3.6	6.7	3.6	6.7
Suarez de Lezo et al[32bc]	60 SES, 58 PES	7.4	19.0	3.3	7.0	3.0	7.0

SES, sirolimus-eluting stent; PES, paclitaxel-eluting stent; p = Not significant for all comparisons.
[a]1-year outcomes.
[b]8-month outcomes.
[c]Angiographic follow-up in only 48% of patients.

ultrasound, demonstration of differences in clinical outcome has been less consistent.[23–28] However, whether disparities in angiographic and clinical outcome emerge in more-complex lesion morphologies is an issue of ongoing study and is particularly relevant to coronary total occlusions.

At present, three comparative trials of SES and PES have been performed (Table 11.3); the first one from Europe is discussed elsewhere.[30] The open-label, multicenter Asian chronic total occlusion registry reported no significant differences in the 1-year target vessel revascularization rates of 3.6% and 6.7% for SES- (n = 396) and PES-treated patients (n = 526).[31] Finally, a modest-sized randomized trial comparing SES (n = 60) and PES (n = 58) in CTO revascularization also demonstrated no significant difference in the 8-month target vessel revascularization rates of 3.3% and 7.0% in the SES and PES cohorts, respectively.[32]

SUMMARY

Until the recent evaluations of DES in dedicated CTO studies, our knowledge of procedural, angiographic, and clinical outcomes following PCI for CTO was limited by the systematic or preferential exclusion of patients with occlusive target lesions from major interventional cardiology clinical trials. Despite these promising early findings in one randomized trial and several observational studies, there nevertheless remains a need for further systematic, prospective evaluation of DES implantation in patients undergoing CTO revascularization.

Given the uncertainty surrounding the development of symptoms in association with a CTO restenosis/reocclusion, the fact that treatment of CTO is usually associated with more extensive stent placement than non-occlusive lesions, and the question whether the improvement in restenosis is offset by a potentially higher risk of thrombotic occlusion, more rigorous clinical investigation is warranted in the field of CTO, not only to confirm the benefit of currently approved DESs but also to evaluate forthcoming novel antiproliferative agents and stent designs in coronary total occlusions.

Despite their common use in clinical practice, neither SESs nor PESs are formally approved by the US Food and Drug Administration (FDA) for the treatment of

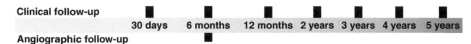

250 patients with de-novo total coronary occlusions 17 sites within North America single-arm trial design

Clinical follow-up

30 days   6 months   12 months   2 years   3 years   4 years   5 years

Angiographic follow-up

Primary endpoints: Angiographic restenosis at 6 months compared with TOSCA-1

Secondary endpoints: Angiographic in-segment restenosis at 6 months; TVF,
                          MACE and TLR at 6 and 12 months; late loss at 6 months
Stent sizes: Cordis Cypher™ 2.5–3.5 mm × 8–33 mm
Pre-and post-dilatation specified with balloon length < stent length
Antiplatelet therapy for ≥3 months

Figure 11.3 Study design of the Approaches to ChRonic Occlusions with Sirolimus-eluting Stents (ACROSS)/Total Occlusion Study of Coronary Arteries-4 (TOSCA 4) trial. TVR, target, vessel revascularization; MACE, major adverse cardiac events; TLR, target lesion revascularization.

total occlusions based on the absence of clinical trials that have rigorously and independently assessed safety and efficacy in addition to incorporating long-term (5 years) surveillance. To resolve these issues, the ongoing Approaches to ChRonic Occlusions with Sirolimus-eluting Stents (ACROSS)/TOSCA-4 trial is a 250 patient prospective, non-randomized evaluation of SES in patients undergoing CTO revascularization using contemporary technique and crossing technologies (Figure 11.3). Clinical and 6-month angiographic outcomes will be compared with an historical control of patients receiving bare metal stents in the prior TOSCA-1 trial (see Table 11.1).

REFERENCES

1. Srinivas VS, Borrks MM, Detre KM, et al. Contemporary percutaneous coronary intervention versus balloon angioplasty for multivessel coronary artery disease. A comparison of the National Heart, Lung, and Blood Institute Dynamic Registry and the Bypass Angioplasty Revascularization Investigation (BARI) study. Circulation 2002; 106:1627–33.
2. Christofferson RD, Lehmann KG, Martin GV, et al. Effect of chronic total occlusion on treatment strategy. Am J Cardiol 2005; 95:1088–91.
3. Buller CE, Dzavik V, Carere RG, et al. Primary stenting versus balloon angioplasty in occluded coronary arteries: the Total Occlusion Study of Canada (TOSCA). Circulation 1999; 100:236–42.
4. Sirnes PA, Golf S, Myreng Y, et al. Stenting in Chronic Coronary Occlusion (SICCO): a randomized, controlled trial of adding stent implantation after successful angioplasty. J Am Coll Cardiol 1996; 28:1444–51.
5. Hoher M, Wohrle J, Grebe OC, et al. A randomized trial of elective stenting after balloon recanalization of chronic total occlusions. J Am Coll Cardiol 1999; 34:722–9.
6. Rubartelli P, Niccoli L, Verna E, et al. Stent implantation versus balloon angioplasty in chronic coronary occlusions: results from GISSOC trial. J Am Coll Cardiol 1998; 32:90–6.
7. Mori M, Kurogane H, Hayashi T, et al. Comparison of results of intracoronary implantation of Palmaz–Schatz stent with conventional balloon angioplasty in chronic total coronary arterial occlusion. Am J Cardiol 1996; 78:985–89.

8. Lotan C, Rozenman Y, Hendler A, et al. Stents in total occlusion for restenosis prevention. The multicentre randomixed STOP study. The Israeli Working Group for Interventional Cardiology. Eur Heart J 2000; 21:1960–6.

9. Rahel BM, Suttorp MJ, Laarman GJ, et al. Primary stenting of occluded native coronary arteries: final results of the Primary Stenting of Occluded Native Coronary Arteries (PRISON) study. Am Heart J 2004; 147:e16–e20.

10. Sievert H, Rohde S, Utech A, et al. Stent or angioplasty after recanalization of chronic coronary occlusions: the SARECCO trial. Am J Cardiol 1999; 84:386–90.

11. Buller CE, Teo KK, Carere RG, et al. Three year clinical outcomes from the Total Occlusion Study of Canada (TOSCA). Circulation 2000; 102:II–1885.

12. Stone GE, Kandzari DE, Mehran R, et al. Percutaneous recanalization of chronically occluded coronary arteries: a consensus document: part I. Circulation 2005; 112:2364–72.

13. Suttorp MJ, et al. Primary Stenting of Occluded Native Coronary Arteries: the PRISON II trial. Presented at Transcatheter Cardiovascular Therapeutics, 2005 Scientific Sessions, Washington, DC, October 20, 2005.

14. Lotan C. Sirolimus-eluting stents in Chronic Total Occlusions (SICTO Trial). Presented at Transcatheter Cardiovascular Therapeutics, 2004 Scientific Sessions, Washington, DC, October 1, 2004.

15. Hoye A, Tanabe K, Lemos PA, et al. Significant reduction of restenosis after the use of sirolimus-eluting stents in the treatment of chronic total occlusions. J Am Coll Cardiol 2004; 43:1954–8.

16. Holmes D. Complex lesions in the e-Cypher Registry. Presented at the Transcatheter Cardiovascular Therapeutics, 2004 Scientific Sessions, Washington, DC, September 28 to October 1, 2004.

17. Nakamura S, Selvan TS, Bae JH, Cahyadia YH, Pachirat O. Impact of sirolimus-eluting stents on the outcome of patients with chronic total occlusions: multicenter registry in Asia. J Am Coll Cardiol 2003; 43:35A.

18. Nakamura S, Muthusamy TS, Bae JH, et al. Impact of the sirolimus-eluting stent on the outcome of patients with chronic total occlusions. Am J Cardiol 2005; 95:161–6.

19. Ge L, Iakovou I, Cosgrave J, et al. Immediate and mid-term outcomes of sirolimus-eluting stent implantation for chronic total occlusions. Eur Heart J 2005; 26:1056–62.

20. Werner G, Krack A, Schwarz G, et al. Prevention of lesion recurrence in chronic total coronary occlusions by paclitaxel-eluting stents. J Am Coll Cardiol 2004; 44:2301–6.

21. Abizaid A. WISDOM Registry: one-year clinical outcomes and subset results. Presented at Transcatheter Cardiovascular Therapeutics, 2004 Scientific Sessions, Washington, DC, October 1, 2004.

22. Grube E, Biondi Zoccai G, Sangiorgi G, et al. Assessing the safety and effectiveness of TAXUS in 183 patients with chronic total occlusions: insights from the TRUE study. Am J Cardiol 2005; 96:37H.

23. Windecker S, Remondino A, Eberli FR, et al. Sirolimus-eluting and paclitaxel-eluting stents for coronary revascularization. N Engl J Med 2005; 353:653–62.

24. Dibra A, Kastrati A, Mehillia J, et al. ISAR-DIABETES Study Investigators. Paclitaxel-eluting or sirolimus-eluting stents to prevent restenosis in diabetic patients. N Engl J Med 2005; 353:663–70.

25. Goy JJ, Stauffer JC, Siegenthaler M, Benoit A, Seydoux C. A prospective randomized comparison between paclitaxel and sirolimus stents in the real world of interventional cardiology: the TAXI trial. J Am Coll Cardiol 2005; 45:308–11.

26. Kastrati A, Mehilli J, von Beckerath N, et al. ISAR-DESIRE Study Investigators. Sirolimus-eluting stent or paclitaxel-eluting stent vs balloon angioplasty for prevention of recurrences in patients with coronary in-stent restenosis: a randomized controlled trial. JAMA 2005; 293:165–71.

27. Kastrati A, Dibra A, Eberle S, et al. Sirolimus-eluting stents vs paclitaxel-eluting stents in patients with coronary artery disease: meta-analysis of randomized trials. JAMA 2005; 294:819–25.

28. Morice MC, Colombo A, Meier B, et al. for the REALITY Trial Investigators. Sirolimus- versus paclitaxel-eluting stents in de novo coronary artery lesions: the REALITY Trial: a randomized controlled trial. JAMA 2006; 295:895–904.

29. de Lezo JS, Medina A, Pan M, et al. Drug-eluting stents for complex lesions: latest angiographic data from the randomized rapamycin versus paclitaxel CORPAL study. J Am Coll Cardiol 2005; 5(Suppl A):75A.
30. P. Serruys, personal communication.
31. Nakamura S, Bae JH, Cahyadi YH, et al. Comparison of efficacy and safety between sirolimus-eluting stent and paclitaxel-eluting stent on the outcome of patients with chronic total occlusions: multicenter registry in Asia. Am J Cardiol 2005; 96:38H.
32. Suarez de Lezo J, Medina A, Pan M, et al. Drug-eluting stents for the treatment of chronic total occlusions: a randomized comparison of rapamycin- versus paclitaxel-eluting stents. Circulation 2005; 112:II-477.

12

Prevention of complications: when to stop–retry–redirect to other therapy

Neil K Goyal and Jeffrey W Moses

Futility of the procedure • **Preventing complications**

In addition to reviewing the different clinical scenarios, wires, and devices to ensure success in percutaneous revascularization of a chronic total occlusion (CTO), it is just as important to understand the limitations of these techniques in deciding when to stop the procedure to prevent potential (severe) complications.

Prior to starting the intervention, the diagnostic films must be carefully studied to determine the appropriate course of action that will ensure the greatest chances of success. The nurses and support staff should also be prepared for the procedure with specialized CTO equipment, including specialized guidewires, catheters, manifolds, and devices such as the Tornus devices, laser, and rotablator. A pericardiocentesis set and echocardiographic equipment should be readily available as well. Preinterventional decisions of vascular access sites, guide support, and methods of anticoagulation are critical. Our routine for approaching CTOs includes dual femoral access with large French (Fr) extrasupport guide in the target vessel and either 5 Fr diagnostic catheters in the contralateral vessel or a 7 Fr 90 cm guide in preparation for possible retrograde approaches. Heparin is routinely used because of its ability to reverse anticoagulation in the case of a perforation. Prior to deciding to proceed with the intervention, it should be noted that there might be situations where the intervention may not be an easy choice. This includes extremely long CTO, heavy calcium burden, extreme tortuousity, and poor distal vessel visualization. Any one of these factors will decrease the chances of success significantly while increasing the chances of complications.

Once the decision has been made to proceed, there may come a point when one must make a decision to stop and try a different technique, stop and retry another day, or stop completely. Factors that play into this decision-making process include (1) futility, (2) complications, and (3) partial success. We will further discuss this decision-making process as it relates to the above factors.

FUTILITY OF THE PROCEDURE

What if the wire will not advance?

In terms of wire management, we generally start with a medium-weight wire such as a BMW or Prowater to interrogate the entry site of the CTO. In situations where the wire will not advance any further and we are sure that we are interrogating the correct entry point, we begin to escalate to stiffer wires with progressively more aggressive characteristics and innovative techniques (Table 12.1), each one of which is described in detail elsewhere. Another approach to increase the support of the wire is to load the wire into a dilating device while attempting to cross the lesion. Frequently, we will use a 1.5 × 9 over-the-wire (OTW) Maverick 2 or a Transit to provide this type of support. Alternative short OTW balloons (e.g. 1.5/6 mm Sprinter) or end-hole catheters (e.g. Quick-Cross) can be tried as well. Other devices that can be used are the Tornus 2.1 Fr or 2.6 Fr.

When escalating wires, a decision must be made about whether to use stiff wires with tapered tips (Confianza series) with or without hydrophilic coating. In general, we begin escalating with non-hydrophilic wires for fear of entering a false lumen. One can start with the Miracle series which are non-tapered yet increase in stiffness from 3g to 6g to 12g of force. If the operator feels that the tip of the Miracle wire is still deflected secondary to inability to enter the lesion, a tapered tip may be more helpful. The Confianza 9g and 12g offer this tapered tip feature. Finally, if resistance is felt in crossing the lesion and the operator is confident they are intraluminal, then one can use the Confianza Pro series, which are the Confianza wires with a hydrophilic coating. Extreme caution should be used when handling hydrophilic wires in these situations as the operator may not have the tactile feedback to suggest the wire is exiting the vessel.

The situation when one would use a hydrophilic wire to initially cross the lesion is when there is a visible lumen. In these situations, a hydrophilic wire may better navigate the bends of the visible lumen/microchannel. Hydrophilic wires that are commonly used for this situation are the Whisper, PT series, Pilot, and Fielder. Another situation necessitating use of these wires in the beginning of the case is the presence of a long or tortuous subtotally occluded lumen before the real CTO. In this case, they can negotiate the microchannels but should be exchanged for a non-hydrophilic wire when the CTO location is reached.

Table 12.1   Dedicated CTO wires and techniques: list of progressive (stepwise) application

- Miracle 3g, 4.5g, 6g, 12g
- Confianza 9g, 12g
- Confianza Pro 9g, 12g
- Hydrophilic wires (when visible lumen present)
- Retrograde approach and entry
- Subluminal tracking and reentry (STAR)

CTO wires offer incremental tip stiffness and wire support. Characteristics such as excellent trackability, 1:1 torque response, and tactile response lead to greater procedural success. Tapered tip design in the Confianza series is also useful.

What if the wire goes offline?

Failure in crossing the lesion may at times lead to the wire going offline into a false lumen. Once a false lumen is created by the wire, a technique to identify the false lumen and allow a reattempt into the true lumen is the parallel wire technique. In this technique, a wire is left in the false lumen and a second wire is taken to probe the true lumen in the area where the original wire appears to have gone offline. By using multiple views, taking advantage of continuously visualizing the subintimal track (outlined by the original wire) and careful manipulation, one can occasionally reenter the true lumen. However, other times the true lumen is not reentered and a dissection plane remains (Figure 12.1). In these situations, one can stop and schedule a repeat attempt in 6–8 weeks. Oftentimes, when the patient returns, the dissection plane is healed and better flow is seen in the true lumen, leading to greater success with the second attempt (Figure 12.2). If one persists and fails to enter the true lumen, a STAR (subintimal tracking and reentry) technique can be used to reenter the true lumen distal to the CTO (Figures 12.2–12.4) Hydrophilic wires such as the Whisper are excellent for subintimal tracking.

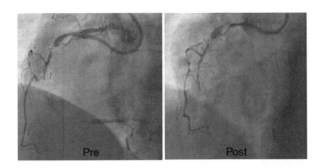

Figure 12.1 Failed attempt at right coronary artery (RCA) CTO leads to vessel dissection.

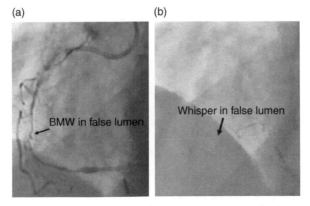

Figure 12.2 The patient from Figure 12.1 is brought back 6 weeks later for a reattempt. Angiography reveals healing of the prior dissection plane with improved flow in the artery. Attempts are made to cross the lesion, and a dissection plane is created, which is seen in (a) with the BMW guidewire in place. Multiple attempts to cross the lesion using a Confianza Pro 12g wire and a parallel wire technique fail. The subintimal tracking and reentry (STAR) technique is used with a Whisper hydrophilic wire (b).

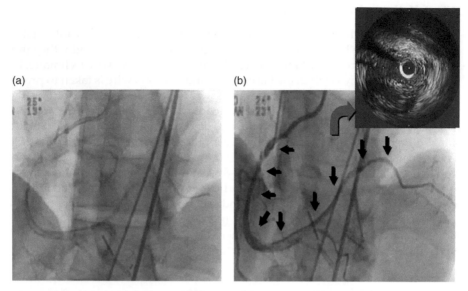

Figure 12.3 (a) Using the subintimal tracking and reentry (STAR) technique, one wire is placed in the posterior descending artery and the other in the posterolateral branch. (b) The vessel post-angioplasty (arrows). Intravascular ultrasound (inset) in the false lumen shows the lumen created by the STAR technique.

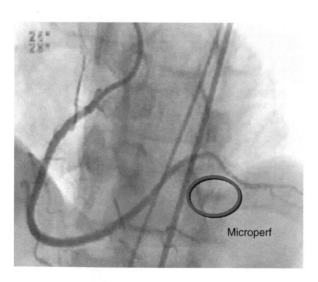

Microperf

Figure 12.4 Final angiogram after five stents and percutaneous transluminal coronary angioplasty of the posterior descending artery and the posterolateral shows a small perforation (microperf) with staining.

Reentry commonly occurs at branch points distally. However, once the true lumen is reentered, careful attention to the distal tip of wire can prevent microperforations, as seen in Figure 12.4. Finally, if one decides not to use the STAR technique, then one can cross the lesion using a retrograde approach. Using a 90 cm guide in the contralateral vessel, the operator can navigate a hydrophilic wire through collaterals into the distal wire with the support of a transit catheter.

Once at the lesion, the hydrophilic wire is removed and the lesion is crossed with standard CTO wires. Once across the lesion, the CTO is dilated and then crossed in an anterograde fashion to deploy stents (Figure 12.5).

What if the wire diverts into a side branch?

If the wire diverts into a side branch when probing the entry point of the CTO, a few simple techniques can focus the probing into the main vessel. First, a wire with stiffer body will allow more directed interrogation without the wire flopping

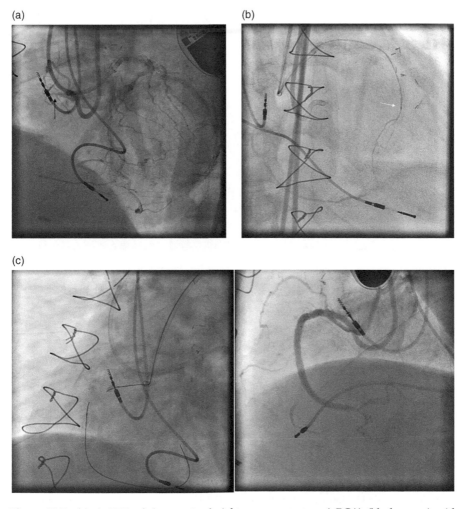

Figure 12.5 (a) A CTO of the proximal right coronary artery (pRCA) (black arrow) with collaterals from septal perforators. (b) A hydrophilic Whisper wire was advanced through the septal collaterals with support from a Transit catheter. Once the Transit catheter is in the perforator, an angiogram via the Transit (white arrow) clearly shows the collateral. (c) Using the Transit for support, a Miracle 3 wire is used to cross the lesion retrograde. An anterograde wire is then passed across the lesion and the lesion is dilated and stents are deployed.

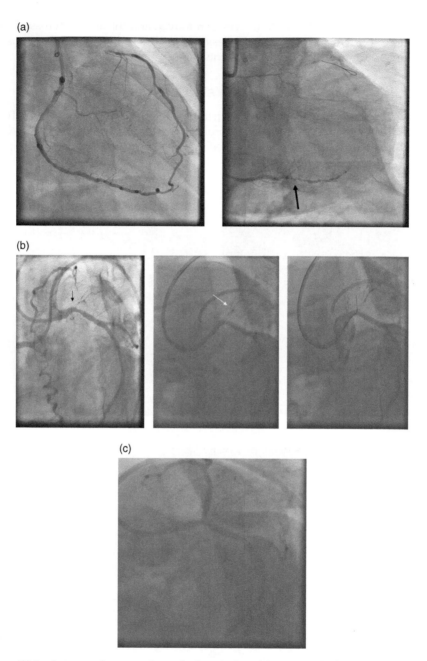

Figure 12.6 Anterograde approach to a flush occlusion of the proximal left anterior descending artery (LAD) guided by intravascular ultrasound (IVUS) visualization of the vessel origin. (a) A flush occlusion of the proximal LAD is seen with collaterals from the right coronary artery. A retrograde attempt at crossing the CTO led to straightening of the collateral (black arrow) and severe spasm with ischemia. The retrograde attempt was aborted. (b) The flush occlusion is seen in the left anterior oblique caudal image (black arrow). An IVUS pullback is performed (white arrow) from a small Ramus branch to visualize the ostium of the CTO. A Miracle wire was then advanced across the CTO. (c) The final angiogram.

out of the main vessel. Small OTW balloons or end-hole catheters as described above can also provide additional support. In order to direct the support, a Venture catheter (St Jude Medical) which has a deflectable tip can help direct the wire. Furthermore, the Steer-it wire is a medium support wire with a deflecting tip that can be used to access the main vessel. Finally, if the main vessel is difficult to identify because of a flush occlusion at a branch point, intravascular ultrasound (IVUS) can be used to locate the lumen. In this situation, a wire is advanced into the side branch and IVUS is performed from the side branch back into the main vessel proximal to the bifurcation point (Figure 12.6).

What if a dilating device cannot be advanced?

In situations where the dilating device cannot advance, there are a few different strategies that can be used. The dilating device that we use as an initial choice, most commonly, is the 1.5/9 mm OTW Maverick 2 balloon because of its favorable crossing profile and the ability for rapid removal and reshaping of wires. However, if this fails to cross the lesion, then the operator should switch to a 1.5/15 mm rapid exchange Maverick 2; we have found that the rapid exchange balloons cross more reliably than the OTW balloons. If this balloon still does not cross, then one can try using an exchange catheter such as the Transit or Quick-Cross from Spetranetics. Then the wire can be exchanged for a more supportive wire such as a Stabilizer Plus or Ironman. If the guide is backing out of the artery during advancement of the dilating device, then an anchor wire with an inflated balloon can be placed in a more proximal branch of the artery such as the acute marginal of the conus branch of the right coronary artery. Some further options include exchanging wires for a rotoblater wire and crossing with rotoblation, eximer laser atherectomy (see Chapters 7 and 16), or use of the Tornus (Figure 12.7), which is available in 2.1 Fr and 2.6 Fr and can be used for backup as well as dilatation (see Chapter 6). After the 2.1 Fr device crosses and dilates the lesion, a 1.5 balloon should cross the lesion right after. A technique that can be utilized as a last resort after multiple unsuccessful attempts to cross over the wire is to advance an end-hole catheter as far as it goes within the body of the occlusion, then remove the wire and attempt to advance the rotablator wire through the last part of the lesion. Given the difficulty of manipulating the rotablator wire (0.009 inch body shaft with 0.014 inch tip), this option could be successful only in very short occlusions, and in general when (1) the most occlusive part of the lesion has been crossed with the end-hole catheter and (2) only the distal cap is uncrossable and (3) is followed by a decent size distal arterial segment.

PREVENTING COMPLICATIONS

Serious complications related to percutaneous coronary intervention (PCI) in CTO include vessel dissection and perforation. Prevention of both is key to procedure success; however, early recognition can also lead to success and prevent further major complications. When advancing wires, one must be cognizant of the path of the wire. Visualization of the wire in multiple different projections can allow evaluation of whether the wire is offline or exiting the vessel. Furthermore, tactile

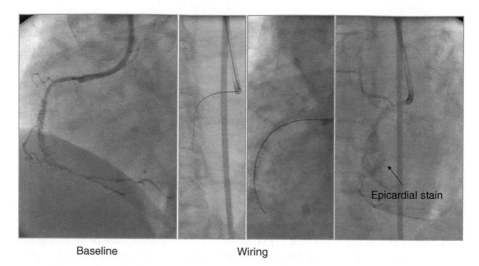

Baseline   Wiring

Figure 12.7   The Tornus device is eight individual wires (0.007 inch) stranded together, made of stainless steel for extra support strength and compatible with 0.014 inch guidewires. Counterclockwise torque is used to advance the Tornus device across lesions.

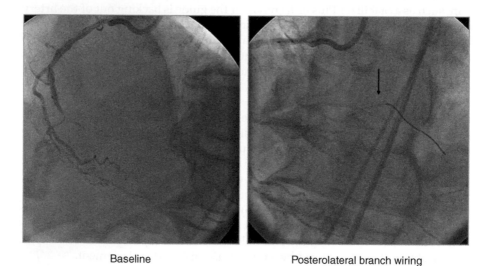

Baseline   Posterolateral branch wiring

Figure 12.8   A complex recanalized right coronary artery CTO that developed an epicardial stain after attempts at wiring. Dilation devices were not advanced and the procedure was continued without evidence of pericardial effusion.

feedback can assist in determining whether the wire is in a dissection plane. By progressive training of these visual and tactile skills, an experienced operator can recognize an offline wire track early and change strategy to a parallel wire technique, thus saving time and avoiding further subintimal tracking.

(a)

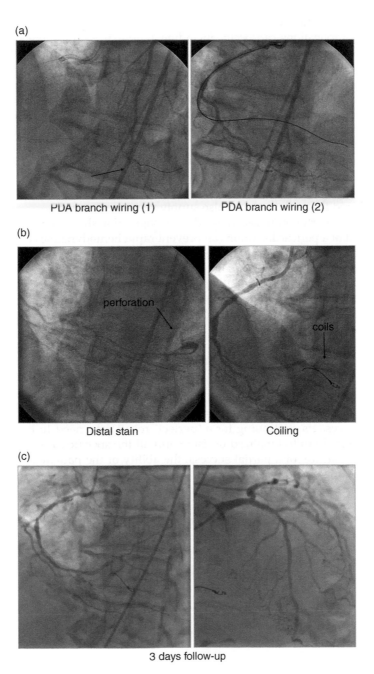

PDA branch wiring (1)   PDA branch wiring (2)

(b)

perforation

coils

Distal stain   Coiling

(c)

3 days follow-up

Figures 12.9 STAR technique in a right coronary artery CTO was performed in a vessel with difficult anatomy. Distal vessel visualization is difficult. During manipulation of the wire distally in attempts to find branches (a), a distal perforation is seen (b, left panel). Immediate treatment of the distal perforation is performed with coils (b, right panel). The procedure was stopped at this time and follow-up angiography was performed (c).

However, if this event is not recognized early, then a number of procedure-ending complications can occur, including wire exit with a large perivascular stain, and vessel perforation secondary to wire, balloon, or device exit. It is critical that devices are not advanced through the lesion until the operator is confident that the wire is in the true lumen. Furthermore, one should avoid injecting contrast media (test injection) distally through an OTW balloon or exchange catheter lumen because such injections can lead to massive distal dissections and perforations. Occasionally, the wire may exit from the true lumen; however, no stain is present or a small 'adventitial haze' is visible. If this has occurred, it is safe to proceed with the procedure if a dilation device has not been advanced (Figure 12.8). However, while proceeding, the operator should pay close attention to the heart borders and hemodynamics for signs of ensuing tamponade. Also, it should be remembered that collaterals can also supply vessel perforations.

If a vessel perforation has occurred, anticoagulation should be reversed. Early placement of a pericardial drain can prevent rapid hemodynamic collapse. Serial echocardiograms can also aid in identification and follow-up of a pericardial collection. An inflated coronary balloon can be used to control flow into the perforation while equipment is gathered to seal the perforation such as coils or covered stents. If devices are not advanced through a wire exit, then a serious perforation is rare (Figure 12.9 (a), (b) and (c)).

Radiation injury and contrast-induced nephropathy (CIN) are two procedure-related complications that are also more common in CTO interventions secondary to the complexity of the procedure and are addressed in Chapter 13.

Partial success

Because of many problems that can arise in a CTO procedure, a decision of partial success vs continuing for a 'perfect' result may need to be addressed. This is a highly individualized decision and all the specific case details matter. The exact 'nature' of a partial success, the ability of the patient to return for a reattempt, the extent of atherosclerosis in other vessels, the need for complete revascularization, the extent of ischemia, the level of symptoms, the global and regional ventricular function, the existence of a surgical alternative, and the related evaluation of comorbid conditions are all important and every case has individual characteristics that have a role in the ultimate decision.

13

Complications related to radiation and contrast media exposure

Masashi Kimura, Eugenia Nikolsky, Stephen Balter, and Roxana Mehran

Radiation exposure • Protection against radiation-induced skin injury • Contrast-induced nephropathy: patients at risk and prevention • Conclusion and implications

Advances in interventional cardiology have resulted in the ever-increasing complexity of percutaneous coronary interventions (PCIs). Successful recanalization of chronic total occlusions (CTOs) in native coronary arteries is no doubt one of the most technically challenging of lesion subsets. During elective coronary intervention for regular lesions, the larger the ischemic insult, the greater the risk of patient death.[1] Angioplasty of a CTO is associated with a similar acute complication rate, although patients with total occlusions have higher 2-year mortality than those with subtotal occlusions. The possible causes for death during PCIs of CTOs may include left main stem artery dissection, arrhythmia, myocardial infarction (MI), and perforation. Procedural success, age >70 years old, ejection fraction >40%, diabetes mellitus, multivessel disease, creatinine levels >2.0 mg/dl, and unstable angina were reported as independent predictors of survival after PCI of a CTO.[2] However, the risk of major cardiac events and death due to radiation and contrast media exposure are quite low compared with those of other complications during PCI.

Although exposure to radiation and contrast media represents an extremely important concern in the management of CTOs, neither of these issues has been addressed sufficiently in the literature, including large prospective randomized controlled CTO trials. The main discussion in the treatment of CTOs typically focuses on the justification of resuming patency of the totally occluded artery, along with improvement in patient symptoms and left ventricle performance, as well as reduction in susceptibility to fatal arrhythmia. However, no prospective study has consistently reported the data on procedural duration, fluoroscopy and cine time, or volume of contrast media, in addition to the status of renal function postprocedure. Furthermore, despite the fact that treatment of CTOs is known to be associated with prolonged radiation exposure and increased volume of contrast media, there are no data on the rates of radiation injury and renal function damage specifically in patients undergoing PCI for the treatment of a CTO. In this chapter we focus on issues related to radiation and contrast media exposure, aiming to increase the awareness of interventional cardiologists and referring physicians to the potential hazardous effects of radiation and contrast agents.

RADIATION EXPOSURE

Restoration of patency of a chronic total occlusion is typically associated with prolonged radiation exposure. This requires a deep knowledge on the part of the operator of radiation physics as well as an awareness of possible radiation injury. There are two principal mechanisms that may lead to radiation injuries in human beings:

1. A deterministic mechanism that signifies massive destruction of cells, resulting in skin injuries and/or cataract.
2. A stochastic mechanism that indicates irreversible damage to DNA, resulting in cancer and congenital abnormalities.

Deterministic effects

Radiation-induced cataracts and alopecia are extremely rare after PCI because the X-ray beams are usually directed from the back of the patient through the chest with no involvement of the head. Radiation-induced skin injury is the most common deterministic effect that occurs as a consequence of a prolonged fluoroscopic procedure. Skin is an actively dividing and moderately radiosensitive tissue. Therefore, skin is the organ that has the greatest risk of radiation-induced injury at the site of direct X-ray beam penetration. Radiation-induced lesions in patients undergoing percutaneous cardiac procedures are typically located on the patient's back. More than 70 cases of skin injuries have been reported in the literature. Retrospective analysis of patients with radiation-induced skin injuries showed significant prolongation of fluoroscopy time in these cases.

Operators need to understand that skin injuries related to radiation exposure are not immediately apparent, and may appear days to weeks after the procedure, necessitating targeted examination for skin changes at 2- to 3-week follow-up after the procedure. Table 13.1 (adapted from Hirshfeld JW et al. J Am Coll Cardiol 2004; 44(11):2259–2282) summarizes the radiation thresholds and biological skin responses to these dosages.[3]

Stochastic effects

Epidemiological data demonstrate a linear relationship between radiation exposure and induction of solid tumors. A slight increase in cancer incidence is observed with an estimated total body absorbed dose as low as 100 mGy (10 rad) or less, whereas a fatal cancer risk increment ranges from 0.04% to 0.12% with an exposure equal to 10 mSv (1 rem). Given the average age of patients undergoing recanalization of CTO is approximately 60 years old, the risk of cancer due to radiation exposure during the procedure is much less than the lifetime cancer risk. Therefore, risk of neoplasms induced by procedure-related radiation exposure is quite low, equivalent to that incurred from 2 to 3 years of natural background radiation.[3]

Table 13.1   Threshold skin entrance doses for different skin injuries [3]

Single-dose effect	Threshold (Gy)	Onset
Early transient erythema	2	Hours
Main erythema	6	Approx 10 days
Late erythema	15	Approx 6–10 weeks
Temporary epilation	3	Approx 3 weeks
Permanent epilation	7	Approx 3 weeks
Dry desquamation	14	Approx 4 weeks
Moist desquamation	18	Approx 4 weeks
Secondary ulceration	24	>6 weeks
Ischemic dermal necrosis	18	>10 weeks
Dermal atrophy (1st phase)	10	>14 weeks
Dermal atrophy (2nd phase)	10	>1 year
Induration (invasive fibrosis)	10	[a]
Telangiectasia	10	>1 year
Late dermal necrosis	>12?	>1 year
Skin cancer	Not known	>5 years

Gy = gray.
[a]No estimate available.
Data derived from References 3.

Attention should be paid to minimizing gonadal exposure to direct beam radiation during interventional cardiac procedures. The radiation dose delivered to the gonads by scatter when the primary beam is focused on the thorax is very small, and the risk of stochastic effects is, therefore, low.

PROTECTION AGAINST RADIATION-INDUCED SKIN INJURY

Preprocedure

Obtaining informed consent regarding skin injury due to radiation exposure is the most important factor for the patient before a CTO procedure. The patient should be made aware of the incidence, risks, and solutions of complications before the procedure. Physician training is also extremely important. The operator must understand the basic principles for minimizing patient dose as well as the equipment's dose-control features. The operator is responsible for conducting the procedure safely and for effectively balancing the benefits of the procedure with the need to minimize the patient's radiation injury hazard.[3]

Periprocedure

Real-time monitoring allows the operating physician to appropriately balance the expected clinical benefits and radiation risks of continuing a procedure.[4] One has to bear in mind that real-time maximum-dose monitoring of the skin radiation dose is problematic.[4] In general, the operators usually convict to the total fluoroscopy time as an indicator for radiation exposure. Although there is a high correlation between the KERMA-area product (KAP), total dose at interventional reference point (IRP), and fluoroscopy time,[4] the latter is an inappropriate indicator of radiation risk because it is not affected by the proportion of cine and fluoroscopy during the procedure. Researchers proposed a study evaluating a complexity index for the assessment of procedural difficulty based on the sum of the integer scores assigned for severe vessel tortuosity in various complex lesions (bifurcations, ostial lesions, and chronic total occlusions).[5] The described index was shown to correlate significantly with prolonged radiation exposure assessed either directly or by fluoroscopy time. These data were confirmed in another study.[5,6]

There is no current commercially available method of estimating peak skin dose while a procedure is in progress. There are, however, some important steps that can be taken to protect the patient from extensive exposure during PCI. The fluoroscopic beam should be limited when the dynamic information is useful, and the number of acquisition runs should be held for an effective and optimal therapeutic procedure. The use of other gantry settings allows distribution of the radiation dose over different skin areas and prevents obtaining a high radiation dose. Furthermore, the X-ray system should be positioned so that the distance from the patient to the image detector is minimized. The beam angulations should be changed during a longer procedure to minimize irradiating any particular portion of the patient's skin. The monitoring person should inform the operator with respect to all of the relevant information about radiation exposure during the procedure.

Postprocedure

Postprocedure dose analysis can provide valuable feedback to aid in both the quality improvement process and the supervision of individual patients. Such analysis is also important if a patient returns for a follow-up procedure or for continuing management if the index procedure was a high-dose one.

Follow-up

Recurrence is common after successful recanalization of CTO lesions. It appears reasonable to redilate coronary arteries that show restenoses and reocclusions. Currently, several attempts are normally made to recanalize the lesion. Operators who intend to treat a CTO should know the patient's risk, radiation dose in previous procedures, previous positioning of the X-ray system, etc.

Patient's prognosis

In one study, short-term prognosis has been shown to correlate closely with fluoroscopy time in a series of 9650 consecutive patients treated with PCI. In this study, mean fluoroscopy time was 18.3 ± 12.2 minutes.[6]

Patients with prolonged fluoroscopy time had increased healthcare resource utilization and higher rates of in-hospital death (3.3% vs 0.3%, $p < 0.0001$), emergent coronary artery bypass graft (CABG) (2.1% vs 0.3%, $p = 0.0001$), stent thrombosis (2.9% vs 1.3%, $p = 0.17$), retroperitoneal hematoma (0.9% vs 0.2%, $p = 0.01$), and contrast-induced nephropathy (CIN) (6.7% vs 4.5%, $p = 0.03$).

By multivariate analysis, prolonged fluoroscopy time was most strongly associated with prior CABG (odds ratio [OR] = 2.39), peripheral arterial disease (OR = 1.91), ostial lesion (OR = 2.87), severe lesion calcification (OR = 2.14) and

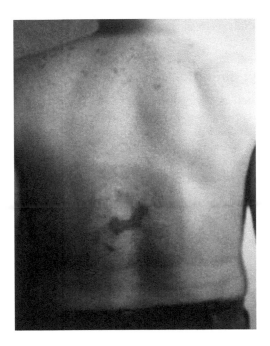

Figure 13.1 Radiation injury. (Source http://www.fda.gov/cdrh/rsnaii.html.)

eccentricity (OR = 1.96), and baseline TIMI (Thrombolysis in Myocardial Infarction) flow 0–2 (OR = 3.71) – all $p <$ 0.0001. Independent predictors of in-hospital major adverse cardiac events (MACE) included fluoroscopic time (OR = 1.04, 95% CI, 1.02–1.06, p = 0.008) and history of MI (OR = 2.82, 95% CI, 1.18–6.72, p = 0.019).

A significant correlation has been reported between prolonged fluoroscopy time and increased amount of contrast media (r = 0.36); it is therefore possible that high contrast volume administration is also related to worse in-hospital outcome documented.[7]

The main radiation safety principle is ALARA (As Low As Reasonably Achievable), which means minimizing radiation doses by employing all reasonable methods. Any possibility of reducing the amount of radiation exposure should be considered in catheterization laboratories. Operators should keep track of radiation exposure, analyze the possible reasons for the prolonged radiation exposure in a timely manner, and carefully weigh the risks vs benefits of continuation of the procedure. A typical radiation injury at the site of beam entry in the patient's back is shown in Figure 13.1.

CONTRAST-INDUCED NEPHROPATHY: PATIENTS AT RISK AND PREVENTION

Intravascular administration of iodinated contrast media may result in iatrogenic renal function deterioration, known as contrast-induced nephropathy. Although the risk of renal function impairment associated with radiological procedures is relatively low in the general population (1.2–1.6%), it is significantly increased in selected patient subsets.[8] CIN-related dialysis in the large PCI series was required in 0.3–0.7% of patients.[9]

Contrast-induced nephropathy: definition and timing

Contrast-induced nephropathy is defined as an absolute ($\geq$0.5 mg/dl) or relative ($\geq$25%) increase in serum creatinine levels after exposure to contrast agent compared with baseline values in the absence of alternative explanations for renal impairment.[9] It typically occurs within 24–96 hours postexposure, with a return of renal function to baseline or near baseline in 1–3 weeks.[10]

In the majority of cases (80%), a rise in serum creatinine occurs within the first 24 hours. Nearly all patients who progress to serious renal failure experience this, with the peak of this rise occurring at 48–96 hours after contrast exposure.[9] Patients with less than an absolute rise of 0.5 mg/dl in serum creatinine at 24 hours are unlikely to have any clinically significant form of CIN.[11]

Risk factors for contrast-induced nephropathy

Identification of patients at high risk for the development of CIN is of major importance. Table 13.2 summarizes the known risk factors for the development of CIN. Unfortunately, only a few of these risk factors are modifiable.

Preexisting renal disease

Preexisting renal disease is the most crucial risk factor in the development of CIN. Its prevalence in patients with underlying chronic kidney disease is extremely high (up to 55%) despite preprocedure hydration and the use of non-ionic contrast media.[12] In one study, CIN occurred in one-third of 439 consecutive patients with baseline serum creatinine $\geq$1.8 mg/dl who underwent PCI.[13]

One has to bear in mind that baseline creatinine is not reliable for the identification of patients at risk for CIN. This is mainly because of age and gender-specific variations in serum creatinine that result in varied levels of muscle mass. To reliably evaluate renal function, an estimation of creatinine clearance should be performed

---

Table 13.2   Risk factors for the development of CIN

Fixed (non-modifiable) risk factors	Modifiable risk factors
Older age	Volume of contrast media
Diabetes mellitus	Hypotension
Preexisting renal failure	Anemia
Advanced CHF	Dehydration
Low LVEF	Low serum albumin level (<35 g/L)
Acute myocardial infarction	ACE inhibitors
Cardiogenic shock	Diuretics
Renal transplant	NSAIDs
	Nephrotoxic antibiotics
	Intra-aortic balloon pump

CHF, congestive heart failure; LVEF, left ventricular ejection fraction; ACE, angiotensin-converting enzyme; NSAIDs, non-steroidal anti-inflammatory drugs.

based on the Cockcroft–Gault formula or the Modification of Diet in Renal Disease (MDRD) equation. As shown in several studies, an estimated glomerular filtration rate (eGFR) of 60 ml/min/1.73 m^2 is a consistent cut-off point for the development of CIN.[14]

Patients treated with nephrotoxic drugs – e.g. cyclosporine, nephrotoxic antibiotics, and non-steroidal anti-inflammatory drugs (NSAIDs) – are also at increased risk of CIN, especially recipients of renal allografts.[15]

Diabetes mellitus

The incidence of CIN in patients with diabetes varies from 5.7 to 29.4%.[16] However, in diabetics with preserved renal function and the absence of other risk factors, the rates of CIN are usually comparable to those of the healthy population,[16] while clinically important CIN usually occurs in a subset of diabetics with underlying renal insufficiency.[17] In one study, CIN occurred in 27% of diabetics with a baseline serum creatinine of 2.0–4.0 mg/dl and in 81% of those with serum creatinine >4.0 mg/dl.[10]

Age

Glomerular filtration rate diminishes with age, and tubular secretion and concentration ability increase the risk of CIN in the elderly.[18] Additional factors increasing the risk of CIN in the elderly include the presence of multivessel coronary artery disease, necessitating complex PCI, coupled with more difficult vascular access. Tortuosity and calcification of the vessels, requiring a greater amount of contrast medium, also increase CIN risk in the elderly.

Volume of contrast media

Contrast media volume is one of the major modifiable risk factors for CIN. The strong correlation between the amount of iodinated dye and the risk of CIN has been well documented. In an early series, the rate of CIN among 228 patients with normal baseline creatinine levels who received a high load of contrast media (250–800 ml) was 4.3%. The rate was much higher (11%) among 54 patients who received >400 ml of contrast agent.[19] According to research by McCullough et al, the risk of CIN is minimal in patients receiving <100 ml of contrast.[9] However, according to others, the relatively safe cut-off point of contrast amount may be as high as 220 ml.[18] Volume of contrast medium is especially crucial in patients with other risk factors. In a study on the diabetic population from our institution, CIN developed in approximately every fifth, fourth, and second patient who received 200–400 ml, 400–600 ml, and >600 ml of contrast, respectively.[17] In the same study, each 100 ml increment in contrast volume resulted in a 30% increase in the odds of CIN (OR = 1.30, 95% CI 1.16–1.46), and there was a significant (p <0.0001) trend towards the increased covariate adjusted odds of CIN across increasing amounts of contrast media.

Type of contrast agents

Iodinated contrast media can be classified by osmolality, including traditional high-osmolar contrast media, low-osmolar media, and alternative iso-osmolar media. Controversy exists as to whether the use of different contrast agents is of any benefit in diminishing the risk of CIN. In a study by Katholi et al,[20] the decrease in creatinine clearance was more pronounced and lasted longer in the group that received high-osmolar contrast media compared to patients exposed to a low-osmolar contrast agent. In a meta-analysis of 45 trials, the greatest increase in serum creatinine after administration of high- compared with low-osmolar contrast media was seen only in patients with preexisting renal failure.[21] Another open-label trial reported that a maximal increase in serum creatinine levels of >25% within a week after administration of contrast media was less common with iso-osmolar agents than with low-osmolar media (3.7% vs 10%).[22] Conversely, Schwab et al[23] failed to show any significant differences in nephrotoxic effect between several studied contrast agents. Despite the uncertainty that still exists regarding the degree of nephrotoxicity of various contrast agents, in current practice low (or iso)-osmolar contrast media are preferred in patients with renal impairment. Further study is warranted to clarify the issue of minimizing renal damage while using different contrast material.

Anemia and procedure-related blood loss

Anemia might be one of the factors contributing to deteriorating renal ischemia. In a report from our institution, rates of CIN steadily increased with decreasing baseline hematocrit quintiles (from 10.3% in the highest quintile to 23.3% in the lowest quintile).[24] Stratification by baseline eGFR and baseline hematocrit showed that the rates of CIN were the highest (28.8%) in patients who had the lowest level for both baseline eGFR and hematocrit. By multivariate analysis, lower baseline hematocrit was an independent predictor of CIN; each 3% decrease in baseline hematocrit resulted in a significant increase in the odds of CIN in patients with and without chronic kidney disease (11% and 23%, respectively).

Other risk factors of contrast-induced nephropathy

Several studies have recognized advanced congestive heart failure (CHF), compromised left ventricle systolic performance, dehydration, hypotension, the use of intra-aortic balloon pump, and several drugs (angiotensin-converting enzyme [ACE] inhibitors, diuretics, and NSAIDs) to be negative prognostic indicators of CIN. In one study, patients receiving ACE inhibitors had a significant increase in serum creatinine after the procedure, compared with patients without such therapy.[18] The detrimental influence of prolonged hypotension on kidney function is well known, and even relatively short periods of hypotension may be hazardous. Intra-aortic balloon counterpulsation may signify a very high-risk population due to hemodynamic instablility and severe coronary atherosclerosis, as well as indicate a role of atheroembolism in the pathogenesis of CIN.[17,25]

Contrast nephropathy risk score

To assess the cumulative risk of several variables on renal function, we developed a simple CIN risk score that could be readily applied by clinicians (Figure 13.2). For this purpose, a total of 8357 patients were randomly assigned to a development and a validation dataset. Baseline clinical and procedural characteristics of the

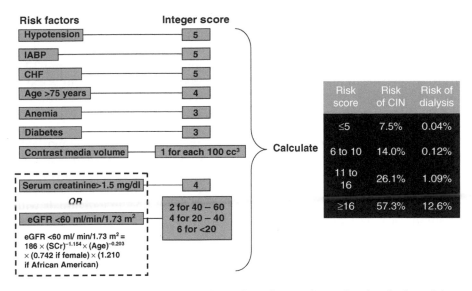

Figure 13.2 Calculation of contrast nephropathy risk score. (Reproduced and adapted from Mehran R, Aymong ED, Nikolsky E, et al. A simple risk score for prediction of contrast-induced nephropathy after percutaneous coronary intervention: development and initial validation. J Am Coll Cardiol 2004; 44:1393–9.)

5571 patients in the development dataset were considered as candidate univariate predictors of CIN. Multivariate logistic regression was then used to identify independent predictors of CIN with p value <0.0001. Based on OR, eight identified variables (hypotension, intra-aortic balloon pump, CHF, chronic kidney disease, diabetes, age >75 years old, anemia, and contrast volume) were assigned a weighed integer; the sum of the integers was a total risk score for each patient. We found that the overall occurrence of CIN in the development set was 13.1%; the rate of CIN increased exponentially with increasing risk score (from 7.5% for a low [≤5] risk score to 57.3% for a high [≥16] risk score, respectively).

The simplicity in assessment of CIN risk post-PCI using readily available information allows us to recommend the risk score for both clinical and investigational purposes.

Prognosis of contrast-induced nephropathy

CIN is an important factor associated with prolonged in-hospital stay, as well as increased morbidity, mortality, and costs. In a retrospective analysis of 16 248 patients exposed to contrast media, in-hospital mortality was almost 5-fold higher in patients who developed CIN (34%) compared with those who did not (7%).[26] In-hospital mortality was 14.9% in patients with preexisting renal disease, 27.5% in patients with preexisting renal disease requiring dialysis, and 4.9% in patients with preserved renal function.[27]

A significant positive correlation exists between fluoroscopy time and amount of contrast media.[6] In the above-mentioned series of consecutive patients with fluoroscopy time >23 minutes, mean amount of contrast media was 398 ± 165 ml compared with 242 ± 100 ml in patients with fluoroscopy time <23 minutes.[6] However, in the same series, there was no significant change in the rates of in-hospital MACE across quartiles of contrast amount (2.5%, 0.8%, 2.6%, and 3.1% in groups of patients that were administered <200 ml, ≥200 to <250 ml, ≥250 to <350 ml, and ≥350 ml of contrast media, respectively; $p_{trend} = 0.33$).

One-year mortality correlates directly with creatinine clearance: 1.5% in individuals with creatinine clearance ≥70 ml/min and 18.3% in patients with creatinine clearance ≤30 ml/min.[28] In the Mayo Clinic registry, in-hospital mortality in patients undergoing PCI who developed CIN was 22%, compared with only 1.4% in patients without CIN.[12] In-hospital mortality is especially high (36%) in patients who require dialysis after exposure to contrast media.[29] One-year mortality correlates directly with creatinine clearance: 1.5% in individuals with creatinine clearance ≥70 ml/min and 18.3% in patients with creatinine clearance ≤30 ml/min.[28] Importantly, CIN is one of the most powerful predictors of 1-year mortality in patients with and without preexisting chronic kidney disease.[30]

Prevention of contrast-induced nephropathy

The unfavorable prognostic implications of CIN make its prevention of paramount importance. Multiple preventive modalities such as hydration, acetylcysteine, dopamine, fenoldopam, theophylline, atrial natriuretic peptide, calcium channel blockers, prostaglandin E_1, hemodialysis, and hemofiltration have been investigated.

Hydration is of primary central importance in reducing the risk of contrast medium–induced nephropathy.[31] In one trial, serum creatinine levels increased by more than 0.5 mg/dl in 9 patients (34.6%) given water orally as compared with 1 (3.7%) given intravenous (IV) saline for 24 hours beginning 12 hours before administration of the contrast medium.[32] In a study comparing isotonic saline with 0.45% saline (each formulation given at 1 ml/kg of body weight per hour for 24 hours starting the morning of the procedure involving the contrast medium), a rise in the serum creatinine level of more than 0.5 mg/dl within 48 hours after administration of the contrast medium was less likely in patients who were given isotonic saline (0.7% vs 2.0%, $p = 0.04$).[33]

N-acetylcysteine has the potential to reduce the nephrotoxicity of contrast media through antioxidant and vasodilatory effects. Recent meta-analyses[34] suggest some benefit from N-acetylcysteine (pooled OR = 0.54–0.73 for contrast nephropathy, defined variably across studies). However, there were also negative studies.[35] More data are needed before N-acetylcysteine can be strongly recommended for the prevention of contrast medium-induced nephropathy.

Several other agents have been proposed to reduce the risk of contrast medium–induced nephropathy.[17] However, there are still many controversies.

Several studies examined the effect of hemodialysis immediately after exposure to contrast media in preventing renal function deterioration in patients with preexisting chronic kidney disease. The results were consistent across all the studies, showing that prophylactic hemodialysis does not diminish the rates of CIN, and may even increase the CIN risk.[36] One randomized study investigated the role of hemofiltration as compared with isotonic-saline hydration in preventing

CIN in a high-risk population. Among patients with advanced kidney disease (mean creatinine clearance 26 ml/min), an increase in serum creatinine levels of at least 25% was significantly less common in patients randomly assigned to prophylactic hemofiltration, before and after the administration of contrast media, than in those assigned to receive fluid alone (5% vs 50%, $p < 0.001$).[37]

Targeted renal therapy (TRT) is a pioneer approach to maximizing the beneficial renal effects of drugs while minimizing systemic side effects using the Benephit Infusion System developed by FlowMedica, Inc., Fremont, CA. This device delivers medications and other therapeutic agents directly to the kidneys via the renal arteries. A randomized, controlled, open-label, partial crossover design trial was conducted in which 33 patients who underwent coronary angiography were randomized in a 1:2 ratio to control or fenoldopam with this device.[38] Compared with IV fenoldopam, selective intrarenal (IR) administration was associated with a significantly higher GFR and renal plasma flow, lower fenoldopam plasma levels, and greater nadir systolic blood pressure.

Sodium bicarbonate has been reported as beneficial in preventing contrast nephropathy in a study,[39] and failed to do so in another. While its utility warrants further confirmation, it is an additional inexpensive option provided that all measures have been taken to avoid volume overload and pulmonary congestion during the procedure. This problem may be accentuated during prolonged CTO cases in patients with abnormal left ventricular ejection fraction or heart failure.

CONCLUSION AND IMPLICATIONS

Recanalization of chronically occluded coronary arteries is no doubt one of the major technical challenges in interventional cardiology. Though the increasing rates of procedural success in the treatment of CTO lesions are encouraging, one should not forget that the procedure is typically associated with a prolonged exposure to radiation and contrast media.

To manage the risks associated with this, the operator must possess a deep understanding of radiation physics, radiation biology, X-ray image formation, and the operation of an X-ray cinefluorography unit. The operator must also be responsible for proper case selection and assessment of procedural risk vs benefit.

In addition, one should not forget that CIN is an iatrogenic disorder, resulting from the physician-directed administration of contrast media. Patients with baseline renal insufficiency and those who develop CIN are at significant risk for morbidity and mortality after invasive cardiac procedures. Thus, a careful risk/benefit analysis must always be performed prior to the administration of contrast media to patients at risk for CIN. Although rare in the general population, CIN occurs frequently in patients with underlying renal dysfunction, diabetes, and the elderly. These risk factors are synergistic in their ability to predispose to the development of CIN. The use of a risk score may identify patients predisposed to developing CIN, and is highly recommended as a tool of preprocedural evaluation of the overall risk of renal damage.

The best and most reliable approach to preventing CIN is to identify the patients at risk, to provide adequate periprocedural hydration, and to minimize the amount of contrast media using low osmolar contrast in high-risk patient subsets. This is especially important in patients undergoing recanalization of CTOs, a procedure usually requiring an increased volume of contrast media. Temporary periprocedural discontinuation of nephrotoxic agents is essential. Repeated use of contrast media within a short period of time (2–4 weeks) should be avoided if possible.

Meticulous assessment of the parameters of renal function and radiation amount should be a necessary part of prospective CTO trials, and these parameters should be an integral part of the safety endpoints in assessing different modalities to treat CTO.

REFERENCES

1. Ellis SG, Roubin GS, King SB 3rd, et al. In-hospital cardiac mortality after acute closure after coronary angioplasty: analysis of risk factors from 8,207 procedures. J Am Coll Cardiol 1988; 11(2):211–16.
2. Suero JA, Marso SP, Jones PG, et al. Procedural outcomes and long-term survival among patients undergoing percutaneous coronary intervention of a chronic total occlusion in native coronary arteries: a 20-year experience. J Am Coll Cardiol 2001; 38(2):409–14.
3. Hirshfeld JW Jr, Balter S, Brinker JA, et al. ACCF/AHA/HRS/SCAI clinical competence statement on physician knowledge to optimize patient safety and image quality in fluoroscopically guided invasive cardiovascular procedures. A report of the American College of Cardiology Foundation/American Heart Association/American College of Physicians Task Force on Clinical Competence and Training. J Am Coll Cardiol 2004; 44(11):2259–82.
4. Balter S. Methods for measuring fluoroscopic skin dose. Pediatr Radiol. 2006; 36(Suppl 14):136–40.
5. Bernardi G, Padovani R, Morocutti G, et al. Clinical and technical determinants of the complexity of percutaneous transluminal coronary angioplasty procedures: analysis in relation to radiation exposure parameters. Catheter Cardiovasc Interv 2000; 51(1):1–9; discussion 10.
6. Dangas G, Balter S, Kesanakurthy V, et al. When is the optimal time to stop complex PCI procedures? An evaluation of fluoroscopy time, contrast media use, and correlation with outcomes. Catheter Cardiovasc Interv 2006; 67(5):796.
7. Mehran R. Environmental issues: Radiation Exposure and Contrast Use/Abuse. Second International Chronic Total Occlusion SUMMIT. 2005.
8. Parfrey PS, Griffiths SM, Barrett BJ, et al. Contrast material-induced renal failure in patients with diabetes mellitus, renal insufficiency, or both. A prospective controlled study. N Engl J Med 1989; 320(3):143–9.
9. McCullough PA, Adam A, Becker CR, et al. Risk prediction of contrast-induced nephropathy. Am J Cardiol 2006; 98(6A):27–36K.
10. Berns AS. Nephrotoxicity of contrast media. Kidney Int 1989; 36(4):730–40.
11. Guitterez NV, Diaz A, Timmis GC et al. Determinants of serum creatinine trajectory in acute contrast nephropathy. J Interv Cardiol 2002; 15(5):349–54.
12. Rihal CS, Textor SC, Grill DE, et al. Incidence and prognostic importance of acute renal failure after percutaneous coronary intervention. Circulation 2002; 105(19):2259–64.
13. Gruberg L, Mehran R, Dangas G, et al. Acute renal failure requiring dialysis after percutaneous coronary interventions. Catheter Cardiovasc Interv 2001; 52(4):409–16.
14. Cockcroft DW, Gault MH. Prediction of creatinine clearance from serum creatinine. Nephron 1976; 16(1):31–41.
15. Ahuja TS, Niaz N, Agraharkar M. Contrast-induced nephrotoxicity in renal allograft recipients. Clin Nephrol 2000; 54(1):11–14.
16. Lasser EC, Lyon SG, Berry CC. Reports on contrast media reactions: analysis of data from reports to the U.S. Food and Drug Administration. Radiology 1997; 203(3):605–10.
17. Mehran R, Nikolsky E. Contrast-induced nephropathy: definition, epidemiology, and patients at risk. Kidney Int Suppl 2006; (100):S11–15.
18. Kini AS, Mitre CA, Kim M, et al. A protocol for prevention of radiographic contrast nephropathy during percutaneous coronary intervention: effect of selective dopamine receptor agonist fenoldopam. Catheter Cardiovasc Interv 2002; 55(2):169–73.

19. Rosovsky MA, Rusinek H, Berenstein A, et al. High-dose administration of nonionic contrast media: a retrospective review. Radiology 1996; 200(1):119-22.
20. Katholi RE, Taylor GJ, Woods WT, et al. Nephrotoxicity of nonionic low-osmolality versus ionic high-osmolality contrast media: a prospective doubleblind randomized comparison in human beings. Radiology 1993; 186(1):183-7.
21. Barrett BJ, Carlisle EJ. Metaanalysis of the relative nephrotoxicity of high- and low-osmolality iodinated contrast media. Radiology 1993; 188(1):171-8.
22. Chalmers N, Jackson RW. Comparison of iodixanol and iohexol in renal impairment. Br J Radiol 1999; 72(859):701-3.
23. Schwab SJ, Hlatky MA, Pieper KS, et al. Contrast nephrotoxicity: a randomized controlled trial of a nonionic and an ionic radiographic contrast agent. N Engl J Med 1989; 320(3): 149-53.
24. Nikolsky E, Mehran R, Lasic Z, et al. Low hematocrit predicts contrast-induced nephropathy after percutaneous coronary interventions. Kidney Int 2005; 67(2):706-13.
25. Nikolsky E, Mehran R, Lasic Z, et al. Low hematocrit predicts contrast – induced nephropathy after percutaneous coronary interventions. Kidney Int Feb 2005; 67(2):706-13.
26. Levy EM, Viscoli CM, Horwitz RI. The effect of acute renal failure on mortality. A cohort analysis. JAMA 1996; 275(19):1489-94.
27. Gruberg L, Mintz GS, Mehran R, et al. The prognostic implications of further renal function deterioration within 48 h of interventional coronary procedures in patients with pre-existent chronic renal insufficiency. J Am Coll Cardiol 2000; 36(5):1542-8.
28. Best PJ, Lennon R, Ting HH, et al. The impact of renal insufficiency on clinical outcomes in patients undergoing percutaneous coronary interventions. J Am Coll Cardiol 2002; 39(7): 1113-19.
29. McCullough PA, Wolyn R, Rocher LL, et al. Acute renal failure after coronary intervention: incidence, risk factors, and relationship to mortality. Am J Med 1997; 103(5):368-75.
30. Dangas G, Iakovou I, Nikolsky E, et al. Contrast-induced nephropathy after percutaneous coronary interventions in relation to chronic kidney disease and hemodynamic variables. Am J Cardiol 2005; 95(1):13-19.
31. Solomon R, Werner C, Mann D, et al. Effects of saline, mannitol, and furosemide to prevent acute decreases in renal function induced by radiocontrast agents. N Engl J Med 1994; 331(21): 1416-20.
32. Trivedi HS, Moore H, Nasr S, et al. A randomized prospective trial to assess the role of saline hydration on the development of contrast nephrotoxicity. Nephron Clin Pract 2003; 93(1):C29-34.
33. Mueller C, Buerkle G, Buettner HJ, et al. Prevention of contrast media-associated nephropathy: randomized comparison of 2 hydration regimens in 1620 patients undergoing coronary angioplasty. Arch Intern Med 2002; 162(3):329-36.
34. Kshirsagar AV, Poole C, Mottl A, et al. N-acetylcysteine for the prevention of radiocontrast induced nephropathy: a meta-analysis of prospective controlled trials. J Am Soc Nephrol 2004; 15(3):761-9.
35. Briguori C, Manganelli F, Scarpato P, et al. Acetylcysteine and contrast agent-associated nephrotoxicity. J Am Coll Cardiol 2002; 40(2):298-303.
36. Vogt B, Ferrari P, Schonholzer C, et al. Prophylactic hemodialysis after radiocontrast media in patients with renal insufficiency is potentially harmful. Am J Med 2001; 111(9):692-8.
37. Heyman SN, Reichman J, Brezis M. Pathophysiology of radiocontrast nephropathy: a role for medullary hypoxia. Invest Radiol 1999; 34(11):685-91.
38. Teirstein PS, Price MJ, Mathur VS, et al. Differential effects between intravenous and targeted renal delivery of fenoldopam on renal function and blood pressure in patients undergoing cardiac catheterization. Am J Cardiol 2006; 97(7):1076-81.
39. Merten GJ, Burgess WP, Gray LV, et al. Prevention of contrast induced nephropathy with bicarbonate: a randomized controlled trials. Jama May 19 2004; 291(19):2328-34.

14

Procedural and technical complications

Masashi Kimura, Antonio Colombo, Eugenia Nikolsky,
Etsuo Tsuchikane, and George D Dangas

Major complications • **Perforation or Rupture** • **Other complications** • **Summary**

Successful recanalization of chronic total occlusions (CTOs) in native coronary arteries is no doubt one of the most technically challenging lesion subsets. New technologies, such as drug-eluting stents (DESs), dramatically reduced restenosis rates in a variety of complex or simple lesions. Similar to non-CTO angioplasty, complications of CTO angioplasty arise from different sources, including perforation, tamponade, guide-catheter dissection, vessel or aortic root, shearing off collateral circulation, distal embolism (due to debris or air), side-branch occlusion, arrhythmia, intramural hematoma, extensive dissection, and subacute vessel reocclusion during or following CTO procedures. In this chapter, we focus on issues related to major technical complications and solutions.

MAJOR COMPLICATIONS

Death and myocardial infarction may occur during percutaneous coronary intervention (PCI) of totally occluded arteries by shearing off the collateral circulation, damaging the proximal epicardial coronary artery or proximal side branches, thrombus formation, arrhythmia, air embolism, or perforation.[1-3] Emergency bypass graft surgery may be required for trauma of non-diseased vessels (such as the left main), side-branch occlusion, guidewire fracture with entrapment, and perforation.[4]

Even with extensive operator experience, periprocedural myocardial infarction may occur in >2% of cases, emergency bypass surgery may be required in 1%, and death may occur in 1% of patients.[5] One of the most common, serious complications during CTO procedures is coronary perforation that may be significantly associated with different types of major adverse cardiac events (MACE) and cardiac tamponade. Coronary artery perforation is of particular significance and necessitates physician awareness, early recognition, and management. Coronary perforation accounts for approximately 10% of total referrals for emergent cardiac surgery, but it is most commonly managed in the catheter laboratory with different types of intervention. According to published data from several large PCI series, the incidence of coronary perforation occurs in <1% of procedures, ranging from 0.29% to 0.93%.[6]

PERFORATION OR RUPTURE

Causes of perforation

Coronary artery perforation represents a disruption of the vessel wall through the intima, media, and adventitia. Risk factors for coronary perforation during standard PCI can be classified as *patient-related*, *procedure-related*, and *device-related risk factors* (Table 14.1). In general, patients with CTO lesions classified as more atherosclerotic and AHA/ACC (American Heart Association/American College of Cardiology) type C lesions are more difficult to treat because they require a higher level of technique and more specialized devices compared with regular lesions.

In terms of *patient-related* risks, several studies found that older age and female gender are associated with an increased incidence of coronary perforation.[6-10] In a multicenter study by Ellis et al,[6] patients who developed perforation were almost 10 years older than those who had no perforation; in the same study, women represented 46% of the patients with perforation compared with 16% of women among patients without this complication.[6]

In terms of *procedure-related* risks, the use of oversized compliant balloons coupled with relatively high inflation pressure to achieve full stent expansion to minimize residual stenosis after stent implantation may cause vessel wall perforation. Several mechanisms may be involved, including overstretching of the most compliant coronary artery segment, a high-pressure jet due to balloon rupture, and outward pushing of a stent strut through the vessel wall. Procedural success and complication rates as a function of balloon-to-vessel ratio and high inflation pressure have been shown in several studies. In a study by Tobis,[11] the use of a high balloon-to-vessel ratio (1.2:1) with a mean pressure of 12 atm for the treatment of coronary stenosis in 60 patients was associated with a mean final percentage stenosis of −8% with one case of coronary rupture. In the same study, usage of a similar balloon-to-vessel ratio with a higher inflation pressure (a mean of 15 atm), applied in the next 300 patients, yielded a slight improvement in the final percentage stenosis (mean −10%), but at the expense of an increase in the

Table 14.1 Risk factors for coronary perforation

Patient-related risk factors	Procedure-related risk factors	Device-related risk factors

Female gender
Older age
	High balloon/stent–to–
	  artery ratio
	High inflation pressure
	Extremely distal location
	  of the guidewire
		Stiff wire
		Hydrophilic-coated wire
		Cutting balloon
		Atheroablative devices
		IVUS in the false lumen

IVUS, intravascular ultrasound.

incidence of vessel rupture and major dissections (3.4%). Finally, in a different subgroup, usage of a smaller balloon-to-vessel ratio of only 1.0 but with a higher mean pressure (16 atm), applied in 162 patients, yielded a percentage of residual stenosis of 1% with a rate of coronary rupture reduced to 0.7%. Likewise, in a series by Ellis et al,[6] the mean balloon inflation pressure in patients treated with plain balloon angioplasty was significantly higher in those that developed coronary perforation compared with those who did not (1.19 ± 0.17 vs 0.92 ± 0.16, $p = 0.03$); the same observation was made by Stankovic et al,[9] where a high balloon-to-artery ratio was associated with a 7.6-fold increase in the odds of coronary perforation ($p = 0.001$).

Coronary perforation as a result of forceful injection of contrast media has also been reported.[12]

Regarding *device-related* risks, there are reports describing coronary perforations caused by guidewire, balloon rupture, intravascular ultrasound (IVUS) catheter, embolic protection device, and guiding catheter.[9,13-15] Recently, stiffer wires for CTO procedures have been developed to dramatically enhance the ability to cross the lesions. Vessel perforation has become particularly important with the introduction of stiff wires for penetrating the proximal and distal caps of the total occlusion. Dilating a subintimal channel may not only result in vessel occlusion or perforation but also may prohibit future surgical grafting of the coronary artery. Special care must also be taken when hydrophilic wires are used due to their propensity for subintimal passage and perforation of end capillaries. These wires may easily enter thin-walled vasa vasorum, which are prone to perforation either directly from the wire or from subsequent dilatations. The possibility of wire dissection can be avoided by meticulous angiography (including dual injections) and observing the path of the wire in orthogonal projections. It is important to recognize that in certain circumstances wire dissection and subintimal tracking can provide a unique opportunity for exiting the occluded vessel proximally and entering it distally via the STAR (subintimal tracking and re-entry) technique.[16] Aggressive guidewire manipulation may result in guidewire entrapment,[4] a complication that can be avoided by never rotating the wire >180° in one direction, and may sometimes be relieved by superselective injections of nitroglycerin or verapamil via the over-the-wire balloon or support catheter.

Incidence of perforation

The true incidence of guidewire-related coronary perforation is most likely higher than reported because some instances remain unrecognized and are self-limited. According to the published literature, the rates of coronary perforation due to guidewire were 0.21% in the series by Dippel et al,[7] and 0.36% in the series by Fukutomi et al,[17] In the latter series, perforation occurred at the treatment site in 12 cases, in a distal vessel in 10 cases, and could not be localized in five cases.[17] In the series by Witzke et al,[18] coronary perforation due to guidewire use was observed in 20/39 (51%) cases of perforation. Of these cases, perforations occurred while trying to cross the lesion with the guidewire in 11 patients (55%), with the distal wire in seven patients (35%), and as a result of wire fracture in two patients (10%). Based on these data, the authors emphasize that the distal migration of the guidewire is an important factor contributing to coronary perforation, and that meticulous care of the guidewire should be taken, especially in patients treated with platelet glycoprotein (GP) IIb/IIIa receptor inhibitors.[18] Several wires are known to increase the risk of perforation. In a study by Dippel and colleagues,[7] 10 of 13 cases of guidewire-induced coronary perforations occurred with the same coronary guidewire (Super Soft Stabilizer, Cordis, Miami Lakes, FL); the wire was subsequently redesigned to enhance flexibility of the distal segment. Stiff guidewires (Athlete and/or Confianza-Conquest, Asahi Intec, Nagoya, Japan) provide the ability to steer, shape, and push, thus allowing accurate advancement through hard fibrous tissue. Because of the high risk of vessel perforation using stiff wires, visualization of the distal vessel is of paramount importance. Hydrophilic guidewires (Choice PT, Boston Scientific Scimed, Natick, MA; Crosswire, Terumo Medical Corporation, Somerset, NJ; Shinobi, Cordis, Miami Lakes, FL) represent floppy wires with a hydrophilic coating; they possess excellent gliding characteristics and reduced friction. However, these wires are known for their limited ability to steer and push. This increases the risk of creating a dissection and/or perforation.[18] These wires, therefore, should always be used carefully and never pushed against resistance.

It is worth noting that the rate of coronary perforation was 2–10 times higher in all published series using atheroablative techniques (directional atherectomy, excimer laser, rotablator, and transluminal extraction catheter) than plain balloon angioplasty with/without stenting.[19,20] The excimer laser probably carries the highest risk of coronary perforation (up to 3%).[6,21,22] However, the device-related learning curve may also explain the higher rates of complications. For example, in one series, coronary perforation in conjunction with excimer laser use occurred in 1.2% of 3000 consecutive patients, but decreased to 0.3% in the last 1000 patients.[22]

In the cases involving CTOs, perforations due to stiff guidewire use are the most commonly observed type, mainly divided into two kinds of perforation: perforation in the false lumen while advancing the stiff wire into the false lumen; and distal small branch perforation after crossing the CTO lesion. In general, special treatment is not required for false lumen perforations because they usually disappear after dilation of another false lumen. In distal small branch perforations, the most important consideration is performing careful observation via angiogram. These perforations cause late tamponade because the operators are often not able to detect them. At the end of the procedure, even in successful cases, final cine angiograms should be carefully taken.

Classification of the coronary perforation

A classification of coronary perforations related to the angiographic appearance of blood extravasation (Table 14.2) was created based on the analysis of prospectively recorded data of a total of 12, 900 PCI procedures from 11 US sites during a 2-year period.[6] Coronary perforation occurred in 62 patients (0.5%). Type II perforation was the most frequent perforation type in this series (31/62; 50%), followed by type III (16/62; 25.8%) and type I (13/62; 21%); the minority of cases were characterized by cavity spilling (2/62; 3.2%).[6]

Table 14. 2	Classification of coronary perforation
Type I	Extraluminal crater without extravasation
Type II	Pericardial or myocardial blush without contrast jet extravasation
Type III	Extravasation through frank ($\geq$1 mm) perforation
Cavity spilling	Perforation into anatomic cavity chamber, coronary sinus, etc.

In addition, other studies evaluated the proposed classification system as a tool to predict outcome and as the basis of management.[6,23–25] Analyses showed that:

- *Type I* perforations rarely result in tamponade or in myocardial ischemia.
- *Type II* perforations have high treatment success rates when managed with prolonged balloon inflation, and commonly have a low occurrence of persistent contrast extravasation, consequently resulting in a low incidence of adverse sequelae.[23]
- *Type III* perforations are associated with rapid development of hemodynamic compromise and life-threatening complications, including abrupt tamponade, the need for emergent bypass surgery, and very high mortality. Notably, *type III* perforation with contrast spilling into either the left or right ventricle or coronary sinus does not have catastrophic consequences and is commonly benign.[24,25]

Management and treatment for perforation

Coronary perforation carries a significant mortality risk. Therefore, management and treatment are quite important and used to be initiated very rapidly. The strategy for treating coronary perforation is best determined by specific angiographic type and clinical circumstances. Based on the angiographical classification, a treatment algorithm for coronary perforations was proposed by Dippel and colleagues (Figure 14.1).[6,7]

If extravasation is limited (*type I* perforation) and due to guidewire perforation, the guidewire should be retrieved to a more proximal location in the vessel. In many of these conditions, prolonged proximal balloon inflations (if tolerated) may help to solve the problem. When limited pericardial effusion occurs, as in type I or II perforation, serial echocardiography may suggest clues to ongoing leakage, as evidenced by changes in the effusion size. Early diastolic right ventricular collapse and late diastolic right atrial collapse are early signs of cardiac tamponade and precede the onset of hypotension.

In *type I* perforations, the management is commonly limited to careful observation for 15–30 minutes with repeated injections of contrast media. If the degree of extravasation does not enlarge or if it diminishes, no further action is required. If the extravasation enlarges, intravenous (IV) heparin-neutralizing protamine sulfate should be given. Direct antithrombin agents (such as bivalirudin) may be more problematic, as there is no antidote for this class of agents. Platelet GP IIb/IIIa inhibitor infusions are not usually used during a CTO procedure. Regarding protamine usage, while its effectiveness and safety have been demonstrated following bare metal stenting, little is known about the risk of protamine administration following DES implantation.

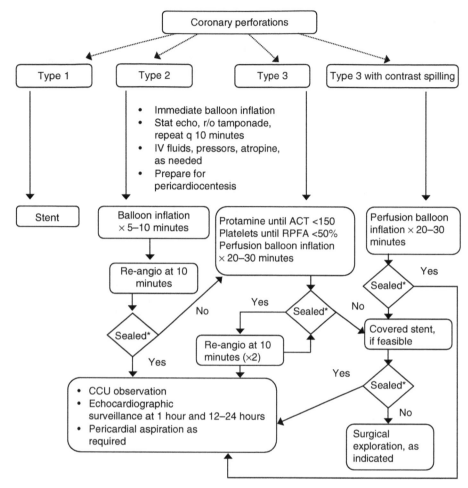

Figure 14.1 Treatment algorithm for coronary perforations. RPFA, Rapid Platelet Function Analyzer, Accemetrics, San Diego, CA. CCU, coronary care unit; ACT, activated clotting time; IV, intravenous. Adapted from Dippel EJ, et al. Catheter Cardiovasc Interv 2001; 52(3):279–86.

In *type II* perforations, the first step in management is placement of a perfusion balloon catheter to seal the perforation.[7,26] Echocardiographic assessment should be performed without delay. Reversal of anticoagulation with protamine sulfate and platelet transfusion in patients who have received abciximab along with urgent pericardiocentesis should be performed in patients with signs of tamponade.[7,17] Emergent cardiac surgery is reserved for those patients who do not achieve hemostasis with these conservative measures.

In *type III* perforations, an immediate aggressive treatment strategy is required, including adequate volume resuscitation, administration of catecholamines, and, frequently, urgent pericardiocentesis. Immediate reversal of anticoagulation with IV protamine and platelet transfusion in abciximab-treated patients is critical. According to the algorithm proposed by Dippel and associates, the treatment of type III perforation should start from the standard balloon catheter inflation at the site of perforation for at least 5–10 minutes to provide time for preparation of a perfusion balloon catheter and to perform pericardiocentesis.[7] Subsequent prolonged perfusion balloon inflation (for 20–30 minutes) may successfully seal a type III perforation or can provide time to prepare an autologous vein, radial artery, or a polytetrafluoroethylene (PTFE)-covered stent. The site of coronary perforation must be completely sealed by these therapeutic modalities and confirmed by an angiogram performed at least 10 minutes following treatment. Intermittent or continuous pericardial catheter aspiration should be employed overnight.[7] Furthermore, the authors recommend in-hospital observation for an additional 24 hours with repeat echocardiography prior to discharge or on the day following pericardial catheter removal.[7]

In limited perforations (types I and II) not caused by guidewire use, maintaining the guidewire position across the perforation site is crucial, and careful balloon compression of the perforation site is usually recommended to limit further extravasation. In patients receiving heparin, reversal of the anticoagulant effects should be considered. Platelet GP IIb/IIIa inhibitor infusions should be stopped whenever perforation occurs, regardless of the severity. In an analysis of the Mayo Clinic PCI database, administration of protamine and prolonged balloon inflation were the most common treatments performed after identification of a coronary perforation.[10] In those patients receiving unfractionated heparin, IV protamine sulfate (1 mg per 100 units heparin) should be given, with subsequent dose titration guided by anticoagulation status to reverse the anticoagulation effects.[17] Reversal of heparin anticoagulation should target an activated clotting time (ACT) of 150 seconds. Protamine may partially neutralize the anti-IIa activity, but not the anti-Xa activity of low molecular weight heparin.[27,28] Reversal of heparin anticoagulation is most easily and rapidly achieved through the administration of IV protamine sulfate.[29] Importantly, protamine has been safely administered to facilitate hemostasis following coronary stent deployment without adverse ischemic sequelae.[30] Administration of protamine and/or platelet transfusion may be reserved for patients who have evidence of a pericardial effusion, and pericardiocentesis should be performed only in the presence of hemodynamic or echocardiographic cardiac compromise.[7]

Specific devices and materials for perforation

Several devices and materials for sealing the perforation site, such as plugs, coils, glues, beads and deployment of covered stents, are summarized in Table 14.3.

Plugs, coils, glues, and beads are usually used for small perforations (*type I or II*) or distal perforations, caused by guidewire, that cannot be sealed with a covered stent. They are more useful for pinhole perforations. Recently, Japanese colleagues have used injections of small fragments of adipose tissue via a microcatheter rather than alien substances such as plugs, coils, glues, and beads. Adipose tissue could be absorbed after plugging the small perforation completely.

After defining the perforation on an angiogram, we recommend reinflating the balloon used in the procedure with low pressure at the perforation site. Dilation with the perfusion balloon should be at the minimum pressure capable of ensuring hemostasis. In general, long balloon inflation (≥10–30 minutes) with 2–3 atm pressure is required to plug the extravascular flow. When the perforation

Table 14.3   Devices and materials for treatment of the coronary perforation

	PTFE-covered stent	Microsphere	Coils	Coils
Company	Abbott	BioSphere Medical™	Abbott	Boston Scientific
Device name	JOSTENT®	Embospheres		GDC® 360° Detachable Coils
Diameter	3.0–5.0 mm		3–20 mm	3–6 mm
Length	12–26 mm		2–15 cm (extended embolus length)	

persists, coil embolization is one of the options for treatment. For the distal perforation caused by guidewire, the injection of the gel foam strips through an infusion catheter is another option.

If the ischemia develops (hypotension), the balloon can be changed to a perfusion balloon. If cardiac tamponade and low blood pressure ensue, pericardiocentesis and drainage with a pigtail catheter are required. One important point to consider is the need to use two guiding catheters in order to be able to control the perforation with the inflated balloon while being ready to advance a covered stent if needed. When extravascular flow is observed on an angiogram despite prolonged perfusion balloon inflation, a covered stent should be used to stop the leakage. However, preparing these covered stents is technically difficult, and the delay of preparation could affect the patient's hemodynamics. The small-size covered stents are compatible with a 6 Fr catheter, but advance more easily and have less chance of dislodging when a larger catheter is used due to the bigger inner lumen and greater passive support.

If a life-threatening perforation occurs while working with a smaller guide requiring the covered stent for sealing, a balloon angioplasty catheter (or stent delivery balloon) should immediately be inflated across the tear in the coronary vessel to provide temporary hemostasis. Another guide catheter should then be introduced from the contralateral femoral artery access and used to cannulate the coronary ostium after gently disengaging the other guide. The covered stent should be introduced into the new guide over a second guidewire and passed just proximal to the occluding balloon, which is then deflated and retracted, allowing passage of the new guidewire and the covered stent for definitive closure of the perforation.[31]

Covered stent device description

The covered stent device was first approved by the US Food and Drug Administration (FDA) in 2001. According to recent reports, the use of a PTFE covered stent can reduce the mortality related to coronary perforation to 10%.[9] The currently available Coronary Stent Graft is a balloon expandable, slotted-tube stent; it consists of two coaxially-aligned tubular stainless steel stents, with an ultrathin microporous layer (75 μm) of expandable PTFE placed between the two stents and welded at its ends, creating a sandwich-like configuration.[31]

Available lengths of the stent are 9, 12, 19, and 26 mm, with diameters of 3.0–5.0 mm. The main limitations of the stent are enhanced propensity for stent thrombosis, which may be diminished by high-pressure prolonged balloon inflation (for optimal expansion, the recommended inflation pressure is 14–16 atm for at least 30 seconds to allow for complete expansion of the stent), IVUS evaluation for proper implantation, and prolonged (6-month) antiplatelet therapy that includes aspirin and thienopyridines.

According to data from a multicenter international registry that studied the use of PTFE-covered stents in either native coronary arteries (77.8%) or saphenous vein grafts (22.2%) in a total of 35 patients with coronary perforation (32/35 patients), arteriovenous fistula (2/35), or large aneurysm (1/35), the deployment of a covered stent was successful in 100% of patients; two patients in this series required more than one covered stent to seal the perforation.[32] There were no cases of procedural or in-hospital death, Q-wave myocardial infarction, or emergent coronary artery bypass graft (CABG), despite 13.9% of the patients having tamponade before the use of covered stent. Based on the comparison of outcomes of coronary perforations in two Milan centers before and after 1998, Stankovic et al,[9] showed that the use of the covered stent was associated with a significant reduction of in-hospital MACE (death, any myocardial infarction, and target vessel revascularization) in type III perforations (from 91% to 33%), but had no impact on the clinical course of type II perforations. A two-center study in Europe reported 49 cases of coronary perforation complicating a total of 10 945 PCI procedures (0.45%).[33] Adequate sealing of the perforation was not achieved by conventional methods (perfusion balloon, reversal of anticoagulation, platelet transfusion with/without pericardiocentesis) in 29 of 49 patients. The first 17 of 29 patients in this series were treated with a Palmaz–Schatz stent (attempted in five patients and successful in only two patients) and/or with emergent cardiac surgery (15 patients). In the subsequent 12/29 patients, perforation was treated with a PTFE-covered stent: in 11 patients, the stent was uneventfully deployed at the perforation site within a mean time of 10 ± 3 minutes (range = 4–15 minutes) using a mean pressure of 15 ± 4 atm (range = 12–18 atm), and ruptures were successfully sealed. Thrombolysis in Myocardial Infarction (TIMI)-3 flow was achieved in all but one case; in one patient the use of the stent was not feasible following distal location of the ruptured site. Thus, in this series, PTFE-covered stents successfully sealed 91% of coronary perforations after other conservative approaches failed. In the same series, pericardial effusion without hemodynamic impairment was identified less frequently in patients receiving PTFE-covered stents compared with those receiving another stent and/or undergoing urgent cardiac surgery (p <0.0001). At mean follow-up of 14 ± 4 months, 10 of 12 patients treated with a PTFE-covered stent were MACE-free. Angiographic restenosis at 6 ± 2 months was found in two of seven patients (29%). Although PTFE-covered stents are considered to be the device of choice in the treatment of coronary perforations, in some situations the use of this stent is technically impossible due to its limitations (limited flexibility and trackability, especially in diffusely diseased vessels) and the distal site of the perforation with a relatively small luminal diameter. In this specific situation, the amount of myocardium supplied by small vessels is rather small, and an attempt may be made to cause distal vessel thrombosis to prevent further blood extravasation and/or tamponade.

Successful treatment of two cases of perforation with intracoronary injection of thrombin has been described by Fischell et al.[34]

Prognosis

For the patient with major perforation in hospital, careful observation with frequent monitoring of the hemodynamics is required after the procedure, and follow-up angiographic examination should be done the next day. After making sure of no adverse findings, the patient can be discharged.

Sequelae of coronary perforations range from none to devastating, and are fraught with early (often instant) and/or late complications. Based on the series by Ellis and associates,[6] a clear correlation exists between the angiographic type of coronary perforation and early complications (Figure 14.2). In this series, mortality and Q-wave myocardial infarction were entirely limited to type III perforations. The majority of cases of emergent CABG and tamponade were also associated with type III perforation (63% for both complications), while emergent CABG and tamponade were remarkably lower in type I (15% and 8%, respectively) and type II coronary perforation (10% and 13%). Other series confirmed the validity of Ellis' classification in relation to early sequelae and treatment modality. In the series by Dippel et al.,[7] clinical outcomes were quite favorable in patients with type II perforation: there were no cases of death or emergency CABG, with only one patient (5.3%) requiring pericardiocentesis. Importantly, these outcomes were achieved despite fairly infrequent reversal of procedural anticoagulation (21.1%), platelet transfusion (15.8%), or the use of prolonged perfusion balloon catheter infusions (26.3%), although the majority of patients (73.7%) received abciximab during PCI. In contrast, patients with type III perforation had high rates of mortality (21.4%), pericardial tamponade (42.9%), and emergent CABG (50.0%), despite more aggressive therapies including the use of protamine (64.3%), platelet transfusion (50.0%), and prolonged perfusion balloon catheter inflation (85.7%). Similarly, in a series by Stankovic

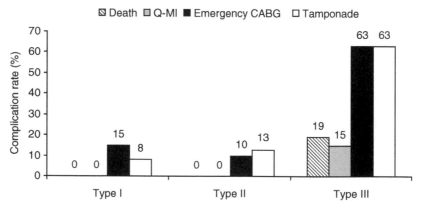

Figure 14.2 Angiographic type of coronary perforation and early complications. Q-MI, Q-wave myocardial infarction; CABG, coronary artery bypass graft.

and colleagues,[9] all cases of in-hospital death and/or emergency CABG (13 of 28 patients; 46.4%) were associated exclusively with type III coronary perforation.

A number of reports have emphasized that pericardial tamponade may develop several hours after coronary perforation. In a series by Ellis and colleagues,[6] there was a 5–10% incidence of delayed (24 hours or more post-PCI) tamponade, arguing for careful patient monitoring, especially during that time period. Delayed pericardial tamponade typically results from a guidewire-related perforation and occurs not infrequently in patients undergoing recanalization of a CTO. In a series by Fukutomi et al,[17] five cardiac tamponade occurred in a total of 25 patients; in 12 patients, the signs of tamponade emerged immediately after coronary perforation, while tamponade had a delayed presentation (after a mean time of 4.9 ± 3.4 hours) in 13 patients who were all treated for CTO. In the same series, a guidewire caused coronary perforation in eight of 13 patients (61.5%), with delayed development of pericardial tamponade. Furthermore, the series by von Sohsten and colleagues,[35] which analyzed 15 cases of cardiac tamponade complicating a total of 14 927 diagnostic and 6756 interventional procedures within a 2-year period, showed that six patients (40%) developed signs of tamponade during the procedure, while nine patients (60%) had delayed tamponade presentation ($\geq$2 hours postprocedure; maximum, 36 hours).[35] Finally, in a series by Fejka et al[19] analyzing 31 cases of cardiac tamponade occurring in a total of 25 697 procedures (0.12%) during a 7-year period, tamponade was diagnosed during the procedure in 17 patients (55%) at a mean time of 18 minutes from the start of PCI; in 14 patients (45%), tamponade presented later (mean time = 4.4 hours post-PCI, range = 2–15 hours). The same series demonstrated clearly that cardiac tamponade related to coronary perforation was associated with high rates of mortality; 13 of 31 patients (42%) in this series died. Mortality was especially high for those patients who developed cardiac tamponade during PCI compared with those who developed delayed tamponade (59% vs 21% in patients).

OTHER COMPLICATIONS

In the past few years, some newer devices (Tornus, Frontrunner, etc) have been approved and rotational atherectomy and the excimer laser have been used for PCI of CTO lesions. Although all interventions share some general management principles, newer devices and new techniques involve some new complications.

Coronary injury due to guiding catheter

In this chapter, the serious complication of perforation is described. However, the most common complication during CTO procedures may be coronary injury due to the guiding catheter since we have recently been able to challenge tougher CTO lesions owing to stiffer wires and new devices. These developments could change the kind of complications we encounter. To give the guiding catheter more back-up force, the choice of guiding catheter which faces coaxially to the ostium of the artery is most important. For instance, most operators prefer to use the Amplatz guiding catheters for CTO procedures to have more back-up. However, the use of Amplatz guiding catheters could injure the ostium of the right coronary artery because the tips could not face coaxially. In such cases, a Judkins right guiding catheter would be fine. If more back-up is desirable, it would be possible to use the anchor balloon technique. During a retrograde approach, we should also be careful about injury to the ostium of the donor artery.

Entrapment of a device inside a lesion

CTO lesions are one of the toughest lesions with severe calcifications. As technology advances, operators have tried crossing and clearing more difficult CTO lesions. In several cases, our group could not advance any dilating devices, although a stiff wire crossed the CTO lesions. In such cases, pushing the device may have resulted in the device becoming stuck. In particular, the Rotablater bar and Tornus became stuck more often. This complication prolongs the procedure time, increases the amount of contrast media, and affects the patient's prognosis. The solution to this complication is:

- advancing another stiff wire forward in the subintimal space beside the trapped device
- advancing the gooseneck snare just proximal to the lesion and snaring the trapped device
- retrieving the entire devices, including guiding catheter and guidewire, together.

During the retrograde approach, it may be possible that the catheter becomes entrapped in collaterals due to severe spasm.

Perforation in collateral artery

In some cases, the CTO cannot be successfully crossed from an antegrade approach. In this case, we sometimes use a retrograde approach, including a controlled antegrade and retrograde subintimal tracking technique (CART).[36] With these new techniques requiring dilatation of a collateral artery, it is possible to cause a perforation in the small collaterals. Coronary artery perforation could cause a fistula into the ventricle if occurring in septal collaterals or tamponade if occurring in epicardial collaterals.

Coronary thrombosis

Recently, the introduction of more specialized techniques (retrograde approach and CART) has increased the complexity of the procedure with the added risk of coronary thrombosis due to prolongation of the procedure and creation of dissection planes. Careful observation in an angiogram (small defect, etc.) can help us to rule out early phase of coronary thrombus. In such situations, we strongly recommended checking the ACT at least each 0.5–1 hour and keeping the ACT at >250 seconds during the procedure. If a thrombus is observed, we should remove it with aspiration devices and avoid embolizing with a thrombus in another non-culprit vessel. If it is impossible to remove it, we should stop the procedure.

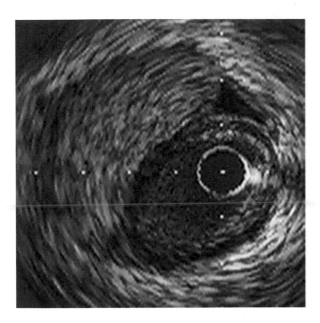

Figure 14.3 Intramural hematoma. (12 to 1 o'clock above IVUS catheter).

Distal embolization is one of the complications sometimes observed after ballooning of CTO lesions. Distal embolization sometimes causes a decrease in the coronary flow, resulting in slow/no reflow. In such cases, the injection of vasodilation agents such as nicorandil[37] and sodium nitroprusside[38] could improve coronary flow, and cardiac markers should not be increased because the distal embolization occurred in the infarcted myocardial area.

Intramural hematoma

When manipulating the stiff guidewire for CTO lesions, guidewires often enter into the subintimal space. Rough manipulation with wire could induce an intramural hematoma (Figure 14.3). An intramural hematoma leads to lumen narrowing at the proximal portion to the CTO site. We sometime need to treat; in rare conditions, intramural hematoma can cause compression of an other vessel. The management of intramural hematoma depends on its severity. After detecting the intramural hematoma by IVUS, if you do not see any lumen narrowing, we do not need to treat. If lumen narrowing extends axially, stent implantation is required. In general, lumen narrowing and axial extension proximal to the lesion do not progress to a critical condition.

SUMMARY

Chronic total occlusion is the last frontier in the field of interventional cardiology. Despite the development of new devices and techniques, certain complications still persist. One of the most common, serious complications during CTO procedures is coronary perforation. The angiographic spectrum of coronary perforation ranges from small-size extravasations with no hemodynamic consequences, to life-threatening events, such as cardiac tamponade, myocardial infarction, and emergent cardiac surgery, and death. Treatment of coronary perforation depends largely on the angiographic type of perforation. Types I and II perforations may be effectively treated with the reversal of anticoagulation and prolonged balloon inflations. Type III perforations should be treated with PTFE-covered stent grafts, demonstrated to be an alternative to surgery. Given the delayed development of cardiac tamponade, a high index of suspicion for tamponade should be maintained for patients with unexplained hypotension after PCI. Once complications occur, careful management and adequate treatment are indispensable. A complete understanding of appropriate decision-making and skills for managing this life-threatening complication should be mandatory for all interventional cardiologists. The most important point is not troubleshooting but avoiding the complication by performing a gentle and careful procedure.

REFERENCES

1. Stewart JT, Denne L, Bowker TJ, et al. Percutaneous transluminal coronary angioplasty in chronic coronary artery occlusion. J Am Coll Cardiol 1993; 21(6):1371–6.
2. Leonzi O, Ettori F, Lettieri C, et al. [Coronary angioplasty in chronic total occlusion: angiography results, complications, and predictive factors]. G Ital Cardiol 1995; 25(7):807–14. [in Italian]
3. Orford JL, Fasseas P, Denktas AE, Garratt KN. Anterior ischemia secondary to embolization of the posterior descending artery in a patient with a chronic total occlusion of the left anterior descending artery. J Invasive Cardiol 2002; 14(9):527–30.
4. Safian RD, McCabe CH, Sipperly ME, et al. Initial success and long-term follow-up of percutaneous transluminal coronary angioplasty in chronic total occlusions versus conventional stenoses. Am J Cardiol 1988; 61(14):23–28G.
5. Suero JA, Marso SP, Jones PG, et al. Procedural outcomes and long-term survival among patients undergoing percutaneous coronary intervention of a chronic total occlusion in native coronary arteries: a 20-year experience. J Am Coll Cardiol 2001; 38(2):409–14.
6. Ellis SG, Ajluni S, Arnold AZ, et al. Increased coronary perforation in the new device era. Incidence, classification, management, and outcome. Circulation 1994; 90(6):2725–30.
7. Dippel EJ, Kereiakes DJ, Tramuta DA, et al. Coronary perforation during percutaneous coronary intervention in the era of abciximab platelet glycoprotein IIb/IIIa blockade: an algorithm for percutaneous management. Catheter Cardiovasc Interv 2001; 52(3):279–86.
8. Gruberg L, Pinnow E, Flood R, et al. Incidence, management, and outcome of coronary artery perforation during percutaneous coronary intervention. Am J Cardiol 2000; 86(6):680–2, A8.
9. Stankovic G, Orlic D, Corvaja N, et al. Incidence, predictors, in-hospital, and late outcomes of coronary artery perforations. Am J Cardiol 2004; 93(2):213–16.
10. Fasseas P, Orford JL, Panetta CJ, et al. Incidence, correlates, management, and clinical outcome of coronary perforation: analysis of 16,298 procedures. Am Heart J 2004; 147(1):140–5.
11. Tobis J. Techniques in Coronary Artery Stenting. London: Martin Dunitz; 2000.
12. Timurkaynak T, Ciftci H, Cemri M. Coronary artery perforation: a rare complication of coronary angiography. Acta Cardiol 2001; 56(5):323–5.
13. Michael A, Solzbach U, Saurbier B, et al. [Bypass perforation by stent implantation: complication management. A case report]. Z Kardiol 1998; 87(3):233–9. [in German]
14. Pasquetto G, Reimers B, Favero L, et al. Distal filter protection during percutaneous coronary intervention in native coronary arteries and saphenous vein grafts in patients with acute coronary syndromes. Ital Heart J 2003; 4(9):614–19.

15. Mauser M, Ennker J, Fleischmann D. [Dissection of the sinus valsalvae aortae as a complication of coronary angioplasty]. Z Kardiol 1999; 88(12):1023-7. [in German]
16. Colombo A, Mikhail GW, Michev I, et al. Treating chronic total occlusions using subintimal tracking and reentry: the STAR technique. Catheter Cardiovasc Interv 2005; 4(4):407-11; discussion 412.
17. Fukutomi T, Suzuki T, Popma JJ, et al. Early and late clinical outcomes following coronary perforation in patients undergoing percutaneous coronary intervention. Circ J 2002; 66(4): 349-56.
18. Witzke CF, Martin-Herrero F, Clarke SC, et al. The changing pattern of coronary perforation during percutaneous coronary intervention in the new device era. J Invasive Cardiol 2004; 16(6):257-301.
19. Fejka M, Dixon SR, Safian RD, et al. Diagnosis, management, and clinical outcome of cardiac tamponade complicating percutaneous coronary intervention. Am J Cardiol 2002; 90(11):1183-6.
20. Cohen BM, Weber VJ, Relsman M, Casale A, Dorros G. Coronary perforation complicating rotational ablation: the U.S. multicenter experience. Cathet Cardiovasc Diagn 1996; Suppl 3:55-9.
21. Bittl JA, Ryan TJ Jr, Keaney JF Jr, et al. Coronary artery perforation during excimer laser coronary angioplasty. The percutaneous Excimer Laser Coronary Angioplasty Registry. J Am Coll Cardiol 1993; 21(5):1158-65.
22. Litvack F, Eigler N, Margolis J, et al. Percutaneous excimer laser coronary angioplasty: results in the first consecutive 3,000 patients. The ELCA Investigators. J Am Coll Cardiol 1994; 23(2):323-9.
23. Del Campo C, Zelman R. Successful non-operative management of right coronary artery perforation during percutaneous coronary intervention in a patient receiving abciximab and aspirin. J Invasive Cardiol 2000; 12(1):41-3.
24. Korpas D, Acevedo C, Lindsey RL, et al. Left anterior descending coronary artery to right ventricular fistula complicating coronary stenting. J Invasive Cardiol 2002; 14(1):41-3.
25. Hering D, Horstkotte D, Schwimmbeck P, et al. [Acute myocardial infarct caused by a muscle bridge of the anterior interventricular ramus: complicated course with vascular perforation after stent implantation]. Z Kardiol 1997; 86(8):630-8. [in German]
26. Maruo T, Yasuda S, Miyazaki S. Delayed appearance of coronary artery perforation following cutting balloon angioplasty. Catheter Cardiovasc Interv 2002; 57(4):529-31.
27. Van Ryn-McKenna J, Cai L, Ofosu FA, et al. Neutralization of enoxaparine-induced bleeding by protamine sulfate. Thromb Haemost 1990; 63(2):271-4.
28. Massonnet-Castel S, Pelissier E, Bara L, et al. Partial reversal of low molecular weight heparin (PK 10169) anti-Xa activity by protamine sulfate: in vitro and in vivo study during cardiac surgery with extracorporeal circulation. Haemostasis 1986; 16(2):139-46.
29. Stoelting RK. Allergic reactions during anesthesia. Anesth Analg 1983; 62(3):341-56.
30. Briguori C, Di Mario C, De Gregorio J, et al. Administration of protamine after coronary stent deployment. Am Heart J 1999; 138(1 Pt 1):64-8.
31. Lansky AJ, Yang YM, Khan Y, et al., Treatment of coronary artery perforations complicating percutaneous coronary intervention with a polytetrafluoroethylene-covered stent graft. Am J Cardiol 2006; 98(3):370-4.
32. Lansky AJ, Stone GW, Grube E, et al. A multicenter registry of the JoStent PTFE stent graft for the treatment of arterial perforations complicating percutaneous coronary interventions. J Am Coll Cardiol 2000; 35(26):A825.
33. Briguori C, Nishida T, Anzuini A, et al. Emergency polytetrafluoroethylene-covered stent implantation to treat coronary ruptures. Circulation 2000; 102(25):3028-31.
34. Fischell TA, Korban EH, Lauer MA. Successful treatment of distal coronary guidewire-induced perforation with balloon catheter delivery of intracoronary thrombin. Catheter Cardiovasc Interv 2003; 58(3):370-4.
35. Iga K, Fujikawa T, Ueda Y, et al. Massive hemopericardium as a first manifestation of coronary aneurysm: successful surgical management. Am Heart J 1996; 131(3):618-20.

36. Surmely JF, Tsuchikane E, Katoh O, et al. New concept for CTO recanalization using controlled antegrade and retrograde subintimal tracking: the CART technique. J Invasive Cardiol 2006; 18(7):334–8.
37. Sakata Y, Kodama K, Komamura K, et al. Salutary effect of adjunctive intracoronary nicorandil administration on restoration of myocardial blood flow and functional improvement in patients with acute myocardial infarction. Am Heart J 1997; 133(6):616–21.
38. Wang HJ, Lo PH, Lin JJ, et al. Treatment of slow/no-reflow phenomenon with intracoronary nitroprusside injection in primary coronary intervention for acute myocardial infarction. Catheter Cardiovasc Interv 2004; 63(2):171–6.

15

Peripheral CTO recanalization and revascularization techniques

Neil K Goyal, George D Dangas, and William Gray

Wire techniques for crossing peripheral CTOs • Device techniques for crossing peripheral CTO • Devices for revascularization: stents, stent grafts, debulking strategies • Case examples

In preparation for a peripheral chronic total occlusion (CTO) the operator should have a plan of approach that is based on preprocedural non-invasive evaluation and imaging of the vascular territory of interest, including arterial segment pressure measurement and duplex evaluation and computed tomographic (CT) or magnetic resonance angiographic (MRA) imaging. Over time, each operator and center will develop its preferred non-invasive work-up based on local availability and expertise with these imaging modalities. With this information in hand, one can appropriately plan the procedure and vascular approach. The important preprocedural aspects of the case include the location of the CTO, and the area of reconstitution keeping in mind important landmarks in the periphery such as the origin of the hypogastric and profunda femoral arteries, as well as popliteal involvement and run-off status. In addition, one can prepare for the use of reentry devices if excessive calcification is noted on non-invasive imaging. Aside from location of the CTO, imaging can also aid in choosing an appropriate vascular access site, and will also limit the amount of contrast media used since non-target vessels/extremity will not need to be imaged. Therefore, the revascularization attempt cannot really be performed appropriately without any proper non-invasive work-up.

When approaching peripheral CTOs in the periphery, one should generally obtain vascular access so as to allow anterograde penetration of the occlusion, since there appears to be less subintimal dissection (especially true in the iliac circulation) with antegrade approaches. Therefore, for distal aortic occlusions, one should obtain brachial access (radial access generally being too distant for the usual length of interventional equipment) if initial attempts from a retrograde femoral approach are unsuccessful. For ostial iliac occlusions, contralateral access is obtained with a plan for exteriorization of the wire once passed through the occlusion to allow retrograde stenting and ease of delivery. For the superficial femoral artery (SFA), anterograde ipsilateral or cross-over contralateral techniques can be used, depending on the tortuosity and calcification of the iliac arteries. A retrograde approach to SFA occlusion is increasingly less common with the introduction of reentry devices, but can be very useful when an antegrade approach is encumbered, although the operator will need to plan a site of retrograde reentry that ideally does not involve much, if any, of the common femoral artery. For patients with combined popliteal and infrapopliteal disease for which an antegrade approach is unsuccessful due to poor targets, a retrograde approach from the dorsalis pedis or posterior tibial vessels via a 4 Fr introducer (but not sheath) and with the use of coronary profile equipment is possible. The operator should recognize that using access other than femoral represents a step up in risk to the patient, owing to the increased incidence of complications in the brachial/popliteal arteries and the end-vessel nature of these alternative access points. When accessing different vascular sites to cross a lesion, snaring and exteriorization of wires may be necessary to dilate and deploy stents at the site.

Once total occlusions are revascularized, final angiography should include the distal vasculature, since distal atheroembolization from these bulky plaques may occur and require management. Some operators deploy distal filter embolic protection devices in these cases, especially in the case of single vessel run-off.

WIRE TECHNIQUES FOR CROSSING PERIPHERAL CTOs

The most common technical approach for crossing CTOs in the periphery involves using a supportive crossing catheter with a hydrophilic 0.035 inch wire. When choosing a crossing catheter, the angle of approach to the lesion and the desire to dissect vs staying intraluminal play into the choice of a catheter. For straight directional access into the lumen of the lesion, a Quick-Cross (Spectranetics, Colorado Springs, CO) catheter provides excellent support. If directionality and steerability are needed, a 4 Fr or 5 Fr Angled Glidecath (Terumo, Somerset, NJ) can be used. Regarding wire choice, like the coronaries, a floppy and steerable wire is used to access the entry point of the CTO. The catheter is then advanced into the origin of the CTO and a decision is made to either penetrate into the lumen or subintimal.

If a luminal approach is chosen, then a straight 0.035 inch hydrophilic wire is an excellent choice, and can be advanced as far as possible until it either crosses the CTO (which happens with startling frequency as long as calcification is not prominent), 'dead-ends', or begins to spiral in a 'barberpole' fashion around but through the occlusion/vessel.

A subintimal approach can then be used, with switch of the wire for an angled 0.035 inch hydrophilic wire, which is more easily prolapsed into a tight curve to track subintimally. As the wire is advanced in the subintimal space, care must be taken to preserve a tight loop (i.e. the same diameter or less as the reference vessel being recanalized); if the prolapsed curve becomes wide, the wire is likely in the adventitia. If this occurs, the wire is drawn back and redirected into a different path, establishing a tight loop once again. If the wire does not have enough support to advance, then a stiffer wire or a 0.038 inch wire can be used. As the wire is advanced past the CTO, the operator should make attempts at reentry into the true lumen.

Options include directing an angled Glidecath towards the true lumen and using a straight stiff Glidewire (Terumo, Somerset, NJ) or an 0.014 inch wire to reenter, advancing a prolapsed wire until the subintimal track feathers into the true lumen, or using a dedicated reentry device like the Pioneer or Outback. Once in the true lumen, the catheter should be advanced into the lumen, and angiography performed via the catheter to confirm position. In heavily calcified vessels, catheter advancement can be difficult; the use of Glide catheters that are spun while advancing can aid in success. We have also modified the tips of the catheters into a beveled configuration, which is usually successful even in the most difficult cases.

DEVICE TECHNIQUES FOR CROSSING PERIPHERAL CTO

Tortuous and calcified vessels in the periphery can make peripheral CTO revascularization extremely difficult. In these patients, the standard wire and catheter technique can fail due to poor guide support, poor wire support, and inability to re-enter the true lumen secondary to calcification. For this reason, specifically designed devices for peripheral CTO can be very helpful.

For luminal access into CTO, the Frontrunner (Cordis, Miami, FL) device can be effective in selected cases. The Frontrunner device is a blunt microdissection tool that is used to create an intraluminal path through the CTO. Over the device, a 4.5 Fr Micro Guide catheter is advanced to maintain the pathway.

If a subintimal approach is taken with any wire or device, reentry can be achieved with Pioneer or Outback devices. The Pioneer catheter (Medtronic, Santa Rosa, CA) and Outback (Cordis, Miami, FL) represent potential solutions to reenter the true lumen from a subintimal space. For SFA occlusion reentry, either catheter will work well; we prefer the Pioneer catheter imaging for iliac/aortic reentry to minimize the risk of perforation or venous cannulation due to the availability of intravascular ultrasound (IVUS) imaging.

The Pioneer is an 8 Fr compatible, 130 cm long catheter that has a tapered tip integrating a nitinol curved needle with a phased-array intravascular transducer (Volcano Therapeutics, San Diego, CA), which allows for two-dimensional as well as color imaging (Chromaflow) of the target vessel (Figure 15.1). The Pioneer catheter is passed into the false lumen over a 0.014 inch support wire, and using IVUS and color Doppler flow imaging, blood flow in the true lumen is identified and the curved needle is advanced towards it. When the needle has entered the true lumen, a second wire is passed through it, the Pioneer catheter is removed, and angioplasty is performed to dilate the track connecting the false lumen with the true lumen (Figure 15.2). A stent is finally deployed to secure the result. A prototype device was used successfully in a few patients, but to date the current mature device has been investigated only in peripheral total occlusions, with a technical success rate ranging from 78% to 92%, with an acceptable safety profile.[1,2]

DEVICES FOR REVASCULARIZATION: STENTS, STENT GRAFTS, DEBULKING STRATEGIES

Once the lesion can been crossed, a decision for revascularization technique must be made. Although stenting has been demonstrated to improve short-term (6-month) patency in the SFA, issues around stent fracture and in-stent restenosis

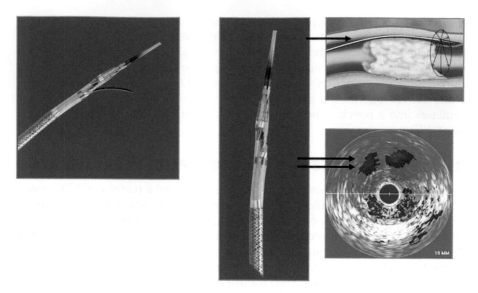

Figure 15.1 The Pioneer catheter allows distal re-entry from the subintimal space to the true lumen with use of a IVUS–based color doppler flow signal.

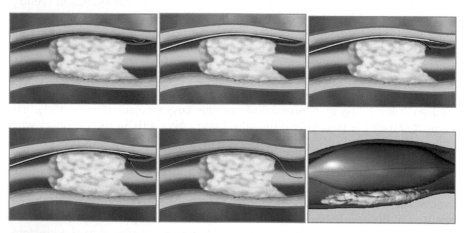

Figure 15.2 A step–by–step process is followed for successful puncture of the distal true lumen with a needle that also allows advancement of a wire through its lumen. This final step is similar for both the pioneer and the outback catheters.

drive operators to alternative strategies. Options for true lumen wire recanalization include both angioplasty and debulking (although no comparative data exist for debulking), as well as stenting, in order to maintain distal flow. Suboptimal outcomes with non-stent adjuncts (i.e. translesional gradient, persistent dissection compromising flow or residual stenosis >50%) can generally be remedied with stenting. For aortoiliac lesions, primary stenting is very effective with excellent long-term patency.[3] While debulking can be performed with the SilverHawk (Foxhollow, Redwood City, CA) atherectomy device (0.014 inch wire compatible system with a rotating carbide blade for plaque excision) or excimer laser (Spectranetics, Colorado Springs, CO) in the SFA territory, it is generally not recommended for use in the iliac arteries where the outcomes with perforation can be catastrophic). If there is extensive subintimal dissection not responsive to angioplasty, stenting can be performed with a wide variety of available devices. If a perforation occurs and is unresponsive to balloon tamponade and anticoagulation reversal, stent grafts can both seal the perforation and maintain a lumen. Since small perforations in the SFA system are generally tolerated well, and seal quickly, the need for stent grafting is generally limited to the iliac system. Perforation below the knee should be managed aggressively, as uncontrolled bleeding can lead to a compartment syndrome (Table 15.1).

The SilverHawk device is shown in Figure 15.3. After delivering the catheter to the proximal end of the target lesion, the thumb switch is switched to the 'on' position, which tilts the nose cone to expose the rotating carbide blade. The catheter is advanced into the lesion thereby cutting the lesion and collecting the cuts into the nose cone. After a pass is complete, the device is turned off, which straightens the nose cone and covers the blade. The catheter is then withdrawn back to the proximal end of the lesion and rotated 90°. The lesion is then shaved repeatedly until all quadrants have undergone atherectomy or until the nose cone is full. The device is designed in nine different sizes for small to large vessels, with different tip designs and lengths (Table 15.2). The TALON study is a multicenter registry investigating the short- and long-term outcomes of SilverHawk atherectomy as primary therapy for femoral–popliteal and infrapopliteal disease; 1-year freedom from target lesion revascularization was 80%.[4]

CASE EXAMPLES

Cases 1 and 2. SFA CTO: basic wire and catheter techniques

In Case 1 (Figure 15.4), we see an SFA CTO that originates just beyond the bifurcation of the profunda artery (black arrow). Distally, we see the vessel reconstituting in the adductor canal well above the level of the knee (white arrow). From the angiogram (Figure 15.4a), we can see that there is minimal calcium in the vessel, surrounding tissues especially in the area of reconstitution. This is important, because this will affect our ability to reenter at the distal site if we enter a subintimal plane. In general, we try to maintain our wire in the true lumen of the vessel; however, in the SFA in particular, it is difficult to stay in the lumen throughout the long CTO. Our access site and sheath support in this case was a contralateral 6 Fr Raabe 55 cm sheath positioned in the ipsilateral common femoral artery (CFA).

An angled tip 0.035 inch floppy Glidewire was then advanced into the SFA CTO with the support of a 4 Fr angled Glidecath. When wiring the CTO, the Glidewire advanced and prolapsed into the subintimal space. The prolapsed aspect of the wire forms a tight curve such that the radius of the curve is smaller

Table 15.1 Peripheral stents

Manufacturer and stent	Delivery	Wire compatible (inch)	Diameter (mm)	Lengths (mm)
Balloon expandable stents				
Abbott OmniLink (Stiff)	OTW, 80 cm and 135 cm	0.035	5.0–0.0	12–58
BSC Express SD (Flexible)	Monorail, 90 cm and 150 cm	0.014/0.018	4.0–7.0	14–19
BSC Express LD (Stiff)	OTW, 75 cm and 135 cm	0.035	5.0–10.0	17–57
Edwards Life Stent Turbo (Flexible)	OTW, 80 cm and 120 cm	0.035	5.0–7.0	11–18
Edwards Life Stent Valeo (Stiff)	OTW, 80 cm and 120 cm	0.035	9.0–10.0	17–36
EV3 Paramount (Flexible)	OTW, 80 cm	0.014/0.018	5.0–7.0	14–21
EV3 Primus (Stiff)	OTW, 75 cm	0.035	5.0–10.0	12–57
Self-expanding stents				
Abbott Dynalink	OTW, 55 cm, 80 cm and 120 cm	0.018/0.035	5.0–14.0	28–100
Abbott Xceed	OTW, 80 cm and 120 cm	0.035	5.0–10.0	20–120
Abbott Xpert	OTW, 90 cm and 135 cm	0.018	3.0–8.0	20–60
BSC Sentinol	OTW, 75 cm and 135 cm	0.035	5.0–10.0	21–80
Cook Zilver 635	OTW, 80 cm and 125 cm	0.035	4.0–14.0	20–80
Cook Zilver 518	OTW, 125 cm	0.018	4.0–10.0	20–80
Cordis Smart Control	OTW, 80 cm and 120 cm	0.035	6.0–12.0	20–150
Edwards Life Stent Flex Star	OTW, 80 cm and 130 cm	0.035	6.0–10.0	20–150
EV3 Protege	OTW, 80 cm,120 cm and 135 cm	0.018/0.035	6.0–14.0	20–150
Covered stents				
Atrium iCast Pre-mounted PTFE	OTW, 80 cm and 120 cm	0.035	5.0–12.0	16–59
Bard Fluency Plus Nitinol-ePTFE	OTW, 80 cm and 117 cm	0.035	6.0–10.0	40–80
Gore Viabahn Nitinol-ePTFE	OTW, 75 cm and 110 cm	0.035	5.0–13.0	2.5–15.0[a]

OTW, over-the-wire.
[a]In cm.

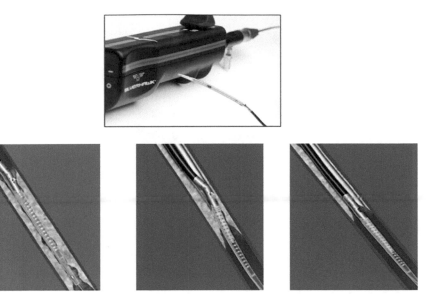

Figure 15.3 The Silver Hawk atheretomy device requires the attachment of a motorized unit (top) to the catheter. A blade is advanced through the plaque and the tissue is contained in a depository.

Table 15.2 Parameters of Silver Hawk device

Vessel size	Device name	Tip style and length	Wire (inch)	Crossing profile (mm)	Working length (cm)
Large	LS	Standard, 6 cm	0.014	2.7	110
Large	LS-F	Standard Flush, 6 cm	0.014	2.7	107
Large	LX	Xtended, 9 cm	0.014	2.7	113
Medium	MS	Standard, 6 cm	0.014	2.7	110
Medium	MS-F	Standard Flush, 6 cm	0.014	2.7	107
Small	SX	Xtented, 4.3 cm	0.014	2.4	136
Small	SS+	Standard, 2.6 cm	0.014	2.3	135
Extra small	ES+	Standard, 2.2 cm	0.014	1.9	135
Distal vessel	DS	Standard, 2.6 cm	0.014	1.9	135

than the diameter of the vessel to ensure that the wire was not exiting the subintimal space. The wire is then advanced with support from the Glidecath in a stepwise fashion. Once the point of reentry is reached, the wire loop is taken out and, using the angled Glidecath, the wire is directed towards the true lumen. After reentry, the Glidecath is advanced into the true lumen, which is confirmed with an angiogram in the distal vessel (Figure 15.4b).

The Glidewire is then removed and an exchange length 0.035 inch Supracor wire is advanced into the distal vessel. After removing the Glidecath, the

(a)

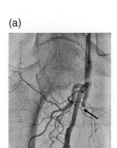
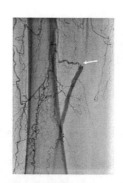

(b)

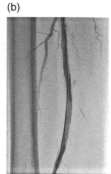

(c)

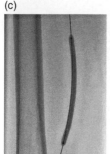
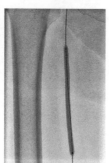

(d)

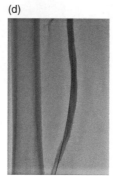
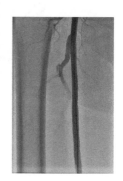

Figure 15.4   Recanalization, angioplasty and stent of a right superficial femoral artery. See text for step–by–step details. a) Baseline angiogram. See text for details. b) Frontrunner device. See text for details. c) Subintimal wiring and re-entry. See text for details. d) Stenting and post–dilatations. See text for details. e) Distal embolization. See text for details.

lesion was predilated with a 5.0 mm × 100 cm balloon both distally and proximally (Figure 15.4c).

A 6.0 mm × 150 cm self-expanding nitinol stent was then deployed distally. A 6.0 mm × 120 cm stent was also deployed proximally, distal to the bifurcation of the profunda. Postdilatation with the 5.0 mm × 100 cm balloon was performed with an excellent final result (Figure 15.4d). Use of these very long stents limits the overlapping segments compared with the use of a greater number of shorter stents; this is thought to be advantageous regarding restenosis/reocclusion and avoidance of stent fracture (although no clinical study has definitively proven these concepts).

In Case 2 (Figure 15.5), we present a similar SFA CTO (Figure 15.5a,b) except that the distal vessel contains a moderate amount of calcium (black arrow). The vascular access and sheath support were similar to the previous example.

The first wire used was a straight 0.035 inch Glidewire inside a Quick-Cross catheter. This was the preferred system because of the short stump in the SFA just beyond the bifurcation. With this system, the wire was advanced intraluminal until the area of calcification, at which point the wire entered the subintimal space. An angled 0.035 inch Glidewire was used to achieve a prolapsed wire tip

(a)   (b)

(c)   (d)

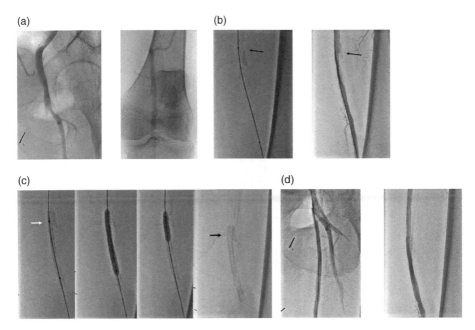

Figure 15.5 Left superficial femoral artery recanalization with a glidewire, angioplasty and focal–stenting. See text for step–by–step details. a) Severe in-stent restenosis. See text for details. b) Filter wire and laser. See text for details. c) Atherectomy. See text for details. d) Final angiogram. See text for details.

to facilitate 'feathering' and reentry into the true lumen beyond the calcified segment (Figure 15.5b).

The lesion was predilated with a 5.0 mm × 100 cm balloon with evidence of persistent >50% stenosis. A 7.0 mm × 80 cm self-expanding nitinol stent was then deployed across the lesion with significant residual stenosis secondary to the non-compliant segment (Figure 15.5c, white arrow). The stent was then post-dilated with the same 5.0 mm × 100 cm balloon to 8 atm and a 6.0 mm × 60 cm balloon to 14 atm with resulting good expansion (Figure 15.5c, red arrow).

A final angiogram revealed excellent flow and lumen both proximally and distally (Figure 15.5d). It should be noted that stenting was only necessary in the area of dissection that had significant residual stenosis.

Cases 3–5. SFA CTO: device examples for subintimal reentry and intraluminal approach

In Case 3 (Figure 15.6), we provide an example of a heavily calcified artery that prevents reentry by the above techniques demonstrated in the two previous case examples. Instead, a dedicated reentry device will be used (Pioneer). This SFA CTO was initially approached with a 0.035 inch angled Glidewire through the sheath. On the baseline angiogram we can see significant calcium both proximally and distally (Figure 15.6a, black arrows). As the wire enters the lesion, we can see

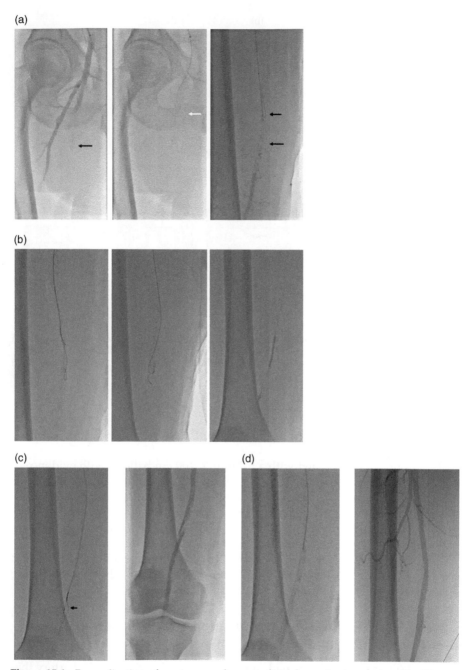

Figure 15.6 Recanalization of a very complex superficial femoral artery lesion. The Pioneer catheter was used for re-entry to the distal true lumen. See text for step-by-step details. a) Baseline angiogram and wiring of left iliac. See text for details. b) Snaring, exteriorization and predilatation. See text for details. c) Bilateral iliac stenting. See text for details. d) Final angiogram. See text for details.

extensive 'barberpoling' of the wire, suggesting it has exited the vessel (Figure 15.6a, white arrow). With the support of a Quick-Cross catheter, the Glidewire is prolapsed into a tight loop, which traverses the subintimal plane as indicated by the straight and narrow path (Figure 15.6a, top arrow in right-hand frame).

Once at the distal area of calcification, the wire begins to loop further out and will not continue to advance in the subintimal plane. At this point, a decision is made to reenter with an ultrasound-guided penetrating device, the Pioneer device. In preparation for the Pioneer, the subintimal space is wired with a 0.014 inch wire and predilated with a 2.5 mm × 20 mm balloon (Figure 15.6b).

The Pioneer is then advanced over the 0.014 inch wire into the dissection plane. The Pioneer needle is advanced into the lumen of the vessel under ultrasound guidance. Through the needle, a 0.014 inch wire is passed into the true lumen (Figure 15.6c, black arrow).

The entry point is then dilated with a 2.5 × 20 mm balloon. Self-expanding nitinol stents are then placed with an excellent final result (Figure 15.6d). Another device similar to the Pioneer is the Outback, which uses a needle for reentry without ultrasound guidance.

Case 4 (Figure 15.7) is an example of the Frontrunner device for recanalization of a right SFA CTO with new-onset critical limb ischemia. Access was obtained in the left CFA and a 6 Fr Raabe sheath was advanced into the right CFA. The proximal entry point is seen with distal reconstitution in the popliteal artery at the level of the knee (black arrow) and patent posterior tibial artery (Figure 15.7a, white arrow).

The Frontrunner device uses blunt dissection in the atheroma to reestablish the lumen. In the images of Figure 15.7b, we can see that the device is advanced and then opened in order to dissect forward. Then, over the dissecting jaws (black arrow), a soft microcatheter is advanced into the new lumen (white arrow). The device maintains itself within the confines of the vessel until the adductor canal, at which point it appears to have dissected outside the vessel (arrow in right-hand frame).

The decision is made to change to a catheter and wire-based system for reentry into the true lumen. First, an angled 4 Fr Glidecath is used with a prolapsed angled 0.035 inch Glidewire. We can see that a wide prolapse occurs (Figure 15.7c, black arrow), indicating that we are outside the vessel. The wire is redirected and prolapsed into a narrow angle (white arrow), indicating a subintimal location. This wire position is advanced to the level of the knee. Then a straight 0.035 inch Glidewire is used to regain entry into the popliteal artery (arrow in second frame from right). An angiogram is performed through a 125 cm long catheter to confirm successful distal reentry.

The lesion is then predilated with a 5.0 mm × 100 mm balloon. The decision is made to use Edwards Self-expanding Life Stents because of decreased risk of fracture and increased flexibility across the joint: 6.0 mm × 120 mm and 7.0 mm × 150 mm stents are deployed distally. Proximally, 8.0 mm and 9.0 mm stents are used. Postdilatation is performed with a 6.0 mm × 100 mm balloon to low pressures distally and higher pressures (14 atm) proximally. Final angiography revealed excellent flow without residual stenosis in the area of the CTO. However, in the posterior tibial artery, an embolized thrombus is seen (white arrow). The vessel is wired with a 0.014 inch BMW and the thrombus is extracted with an

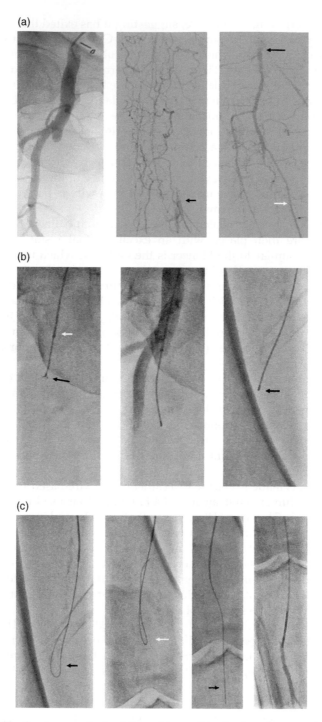

Figure 15.7 The frontrunner device followed by a glidewire–based penetration to the true lumen was used in this case. See text for step–by–step details. a) Baseline angiogram from bilateral access. b) Attempts at wiring. c) Successful wiring and stenting.

(d)

(e)

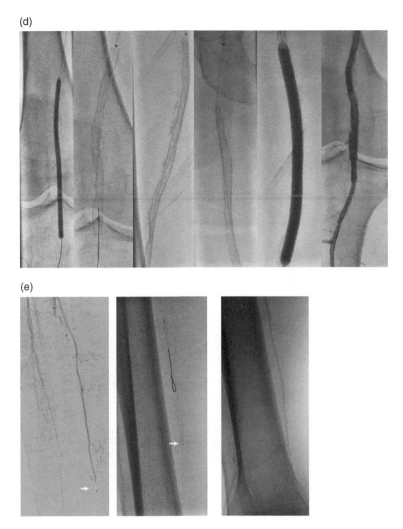

Figure 15.7 (Continued) Angioplasty and stents of the SFA were performed, with 2–vessel run–off below the knee.

aspiration catheter (Pronto). Final angiography reveals return of flow to the posterior tibial artery (Figure 15.7e).

Case 5 (Figure 15.8) is a diabetic with severe coronary artery disease status post (s/p) multiple stents, brachytherapy, and drug-eluting stents) with severe incapacitating claudication who has been refusing surgery. Angiography indicates occlusive in-stent restenosis throughout the four left SFA stents (Figure 15.8a, left side); the occlusion starts proximal to the stent edge with popliteal artery reconstitution via collaterals with three-vessel run-off (Figure 15.8a, right side). Contralateral access with an 8 Fr Raabe sheath was obtained and the left femoral artery was

(a)

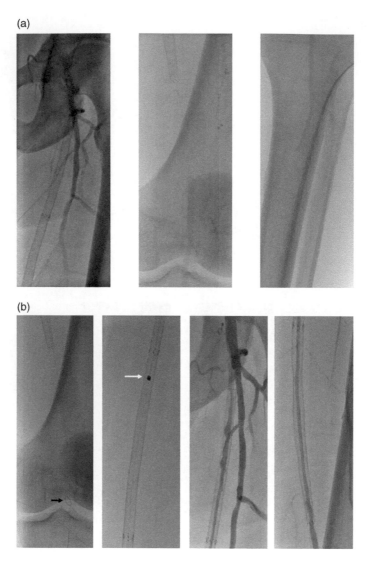

(b)

Figure 15.8 Recanalization of an occlusive in-stent restenosis lesion was achieved and laser was initially used for debulking. See text for step–by–step details. a) Baseline angiogram. b) Attempts at wiring. c) Failed wiring. d) Additional angiography. e) Subintimal wiring and Pioneer re-entry. f) Predilatation. g) Larger predilatation. h) Stent deployment. i) Final angiogram.

selectively engaged; anticoagulation was achieved with 5000 units of heparin (activated clotting time [ACT] = 280 seconds). A 5 Fr multipurpose catheter was used for support and a 0.035 inch straight, stiff shaft, Glidewide was advanced through the lesion and then exchanged for a Supracor wire. An EX-filterWire was advanced next to it and opened in the middle of the popliteal artery; the

(c)

(d)

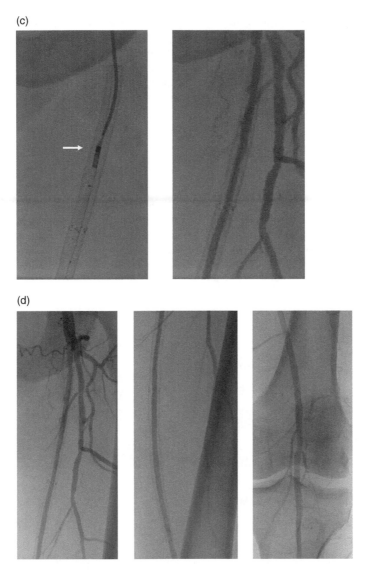

Figure 15.8   (Continued) Under distal embolic protection, further debulking was performed with SilverHawk atherectomy.

support wire was removed and the rest of the case was performed over the filter-wire (Figure 15.8b, left side, black arrow). First, laser atherectomy was performed (Figure 15.8b, white arrow), with improvement in flow and visualization of in-stent restenosis from the proximal to distal edge of the stents (Figure 15.8b, right two frames). An LX-type SilverHawk catheter was used for sequential atherectomy cuts (Figure 15.8c, white arrow). Special care was taken to initiate atherectomy within the patent proximal stent area in order to avoid possible interference with the stent edges; the same care was taken around the overlapped stent segments and the distal stent edge. Four circumferential cuts were performed within each stent; the catheter had to be removed to empty the excised material periodically (every 3–4 runs). The filter was retrieved after completion of a total of 29 atherectomy runs, and the final angiographic result was excellent, with absence of any dissection; accordingly, no new stent implantation was necessary (Figure 15.8d frames).

Cases 6–8: Aortoiliac CTOs

Case 6 (Figure 15.9) is a left common iliac CTO with reconstitution just above the left hypogastric artery. A cross-over anterograde approach is taken from vascular access in the right CFA. Vascular access is also obtained in the left CFA for exteriorization and delivery of devices into the lesion. First an abdominal aortogram displays the CTO in the left common iliac artery. A 5 Fr OmniFlush catheter is used to approach the origin of the CTO and a 0.035 inch angled soft Glidewire is advanced through the CTO (Figure 15.9a).

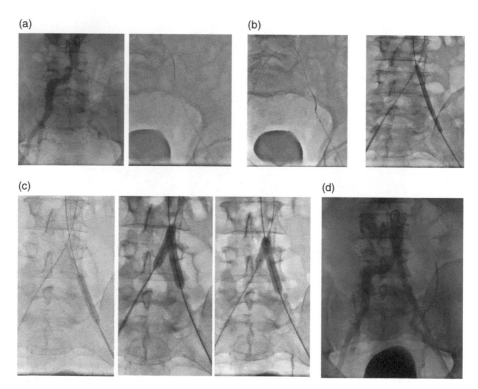

Figure 15.9 Recanalization of a left common iliac artery with antegrade approach via the confuelateral femoral artery access. See text for step–by–step details.

The OmniFlush catheter is then advanced across the CTO. A Supracor wire is then advanced into the right CFA, snared with a 10 mm microsnare, and exteriorized via the left CFA (Figure 15.9b).

After predilatation, 8.0 mm × 37 mm and 7.0 mm × 27 mm Express balloon-expandable stents are deployed in the left common iliac (CI) and right CI, respectively. A second 7.0 mm × 37 mm stent is placed in the left CI and final kissing balloon inflation is performed (Figure 15.9c). The final angiographic result is shown in Figure 15.9d.

Case 7 (Figure 15.10) is a complicated aortoiliac CTO. Pre-cath MRA displayed an occluded distal aorta with collaterals. Sheaths were introduced into the left brachial artery, left CFA, and right CFA. Angiograms from the CFA sites revealed a diseased right common iliac artery with distal aorta occlusion and left common iliac artery occlusion (Figure 15.10a, left side). The left transfemoral angiogram shows reconstitution of the left iliac CTO above the hypogastric artery (Figure 15.10a, right side).

Using a 5 Fr angled Glidecath inside a 6 Fr Raabe sheath and an angled 0.035 inch soft Glidewire, the left common iliac occlusion was crossed anterograde. The wire was then snared and exteriorized through the left common femoral sheath (Figure 15.10b, white arrow). An angled Glidecath was then advanced into the distal aorta occlusion. Attempts at retrograde penetration of the distal aorta with angled and straight wires failed to enter the true lumen (Figure 15.10b, black arrow).

Therefore, the brachial access site was used to penetrate the occlusion anterograde with a 0.018 inch/0.035 inch TAD wire. The aortic CTO was dilated with a 7.0 mm × 40 mm balloon to 6 atm (Figure 15.10c, left side). Once the aortic CTO was dilated, two Supracor wires were easily passed via both access sites across the iliac arteries into the aorta. IVUS was performed to assess the disease and vessel size in the distal aorta (Figure 15.10c, middle). Two 7.0 mm × 57 mm balloon-expandable stents were then deployed in a Y-technique with excellent final angiographic result (Figure 15.10c, right side).

Case 8 (Figure 15.11) is a tight common iliac artery CTO in a highly symptomatic patient. The occlusion is visualized with an OmniFlush catheter advanced via a left femoral arterial access (Figure 15.11a), which was then directed towards the stump and a 0.035 inch angled Glidewire was advanced inside the occlusion (Figure 15.11b). However, neither the catheter nor the wire could be advanced far, and additional advancement threatened dislodgement of the entire system in the aorta (Figure 15.11c). Contralateral access from the right CFA was then ascertained, and selective angiogram showed the end of the iliac occlusion to be at the origin of the hypogastric artery (Figure 15.11d). Advancement of a Glidewire in a retrograde fashion was unsuccessful, as it was ending up medially to the stump; a Pioneer catheter (Medtronic, Santa Rosa, CA) was then advanced over the wire at the farthest possible subintimal position (Figure 15.11e). Under IVUS guidance (in this case also under angiographic guidance since the stump was easily visualized next to the transducer in Figure 15.11e), the device needle was externalized towards the aorta and an 0.014 inch wire was successfully passed through the needle lumen into the distal abdominal aorta, the Pioneer catheter was removed, and dilation was performed with a 3.0/40 mm balloon (Figure 15.11f), followed by exchange of the wire with a stiffer Supracor, and repeat dilation with a long 6.0/80 mm balloon (Figure 15.11g). Following deployment of two 10/80 mm

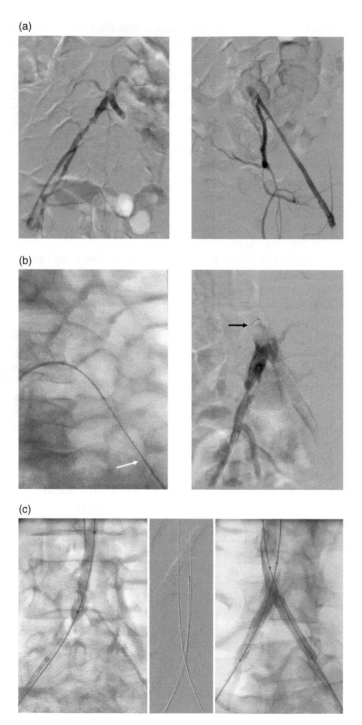

Figure 15.10   Complicated occlusion of distal aorta and left common iliac artery. Bilateral femoral as well as brachial access was used. See text for step–by–step details.

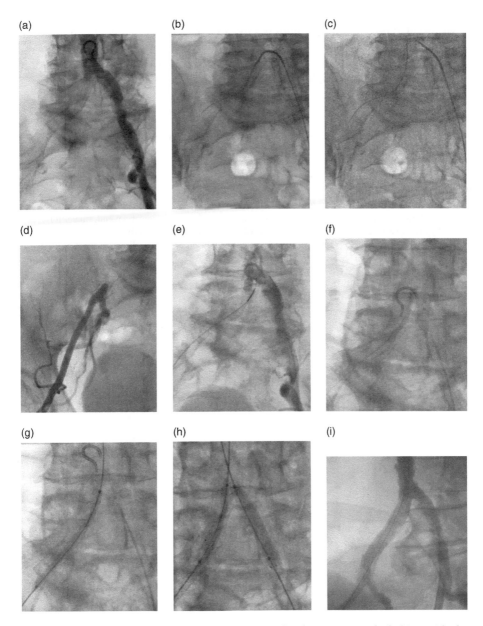

Figure 15.11 Right common iliac artery CTO recanalized in a retrograde fashion with the Pioneer catheter. See text for step–by–step details.

self-expanding stents in a 'kissing fashion,' a kissing balloon inflation was performed at the aortic bifurcation (Figure 15.11h), and an excellent angiographic result was achieved (Figure 15.11i). Of note, self-expanding stents were preferred to avoid possible aortoiliac rupture from the forceful deployment of balloon-expandable stents with high pressure at the site of the deep subintimal track.

REFERENCES

1. Shaw MB, DeNunzio M, Hinwood D, et al. The results of subintimal angioplasty in a district general hospital. Eur J Vasc Endovasc Surg 2002; 24:524–7.
2. Treiman GS, Whiting JH, Treiman RL, et al. Treatment of limb-threatening ischemia with percutaneous intentional extraluminal recanalization: a preliminary evaluation. J Vasc Surg 2003; 38:29–35.
3. Hirsch AT, Haskal ZJ, Hertzer NR, et al. ACC/AHA 2005 Practice Guidelines for the management of patients with peripheral arterial disease (lower extremity, renal, mesenteric, and abdominal aortic): executive summary: a collaborative report from the American Association for Vascular Surgery/Society of Vascular Surgery, Society for Cardiovascular Angiography and Interventions, Society for Vascular Medicine and Biology, Society of Interventional Radiology, and the ACC/AHA Task Force on Practice Guidelines (Writing Committee to Develop Guidelines for the Management of Patients With Peripheral Arterial Disease). Circulation 2006; 113:1474–547.
4. Website (accessed November 15, 2006): http://investor.foxhollowtech.com/ReleaseDetail. cfm?ReleaseID=5166357. Oral presentation by Dr Venkatesh Ramaiah, Society for Vascular Surgery, 2005 Annual Meeting.

16

Role of excimer laser

Steven R Bailey

Chronic total occlusions (CTOs) of coronary and peripheral arteries are increasingly encountered in clinical practice as the procedural complexity increases and more patients are referred later in their clinical course for attempted revascularization. Previous authors in this text have discussed the pathology of CTOs, but there are special considerations in the (`uncrossable`) lesions that deserve special mention. While limited pathological studies of coronary arteries are available, the few studies that are reported in the literature[1-3] stress two specific findings: (1) the presence of calcification and (2) the size and number of capillaries and arterioles present in the CTO. In peripheral vessels, the pathological findings probably include a third pathological process: thrombus in various stages of organization. Examples of pathological findings that have an impact on the use of laser energy for atherectomy are seen in Figure 16.1. Note that many lesions will include a variety of pathological abnormalities along the length of a single lesion. The longer the lesion, the more likely that multiple pathological changes will be present. Thrombus seems to play a more important role in the small vessels found below the popliteal artery in patients with chronic limb ischemia.[4]

Given the disparity in the pathology and technical approaches, it is important to consider uncrossable coronary lesions and peripheral chronic total occlusive lesions separately.

ROLE OF LASER IN CORONARY OCCLUSIONS

Laser therapy, in theory, is uniquely capable of approaching these complex lesions.[5] The excimer laser, or the use of the *excited dimer* of xenon chloride, is the only system currently used clinically for vascular applications. Other laser systems operate in the longer, infrared wavelengths, whereas the excimer laser has a wavelength of 308 nm in the ultraviolet spectra. Korovin[6] demonstrated that the peak absorbance of atherosclerotic plaque is in the ultraviolet spectra at 240

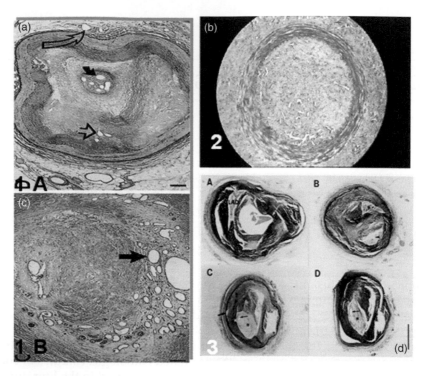

Figure 16.1   Chronic total occlusions have multiple pathological appearances. The spectrum of pathology may vary from firmly fibrotic, to densely calcified, to a vessel with multiple channels. (a and c, reproduced from Srivast et al,[1] with permission; b, reproduced from with permission; d, reproduced from Katsuragawa et al,[2] with permission.)

and 280 nm, which is close to the 308 nm wavelength emitted by the excimer laser. The laser has three mechanisms of tissue and thrombus ablation:[7–12]

- photochemical, in which light breaks chemical bonds
- photothermal, which occurs when the laser energy produces heat
- photomechanical, when light directly produces mechanical energy.

The combination of these three mechanisms might increase the chances of success for laser therapy of CTOs by treating fibro-occlusive lesions, ablating thrombus, and mechanically fracturing calcium. Utilizing all three mechanisms is important when using the laser to cross CTO lesions that allowed an initial wire pass but could not subsequently be crossed with conventional balloon technology. This technology differs from rotational atherectomy in that small particles are not generated, which may be more problematic in limited outflow situations. The laser system is also more likely to 'track the wire' when advanced through tortuous vessels, decreasing the risk of perforations. Finally, the laser system will often decrease the procedure time compared with prolonged balloon-based procedures by decreasing the time and equipment required to cross the lesion. Clinical outcomes are dependent upon recanalizing coronary CTO. In the TOAST-GISI study of 390 lesions, Olivari et al[13] demonstrated that failure to reopen a CTO resulted in a 7-fold higher risk of myocardial infarction (MI) and a 5-fold higher rate of coronary artery bypass graft (CABG) at 1 year. These data are similar to other studies evaluating late outcome after failed attempts to open CTOs.

CHRONIC CORONARY OCCLUSIONS

In approaching chronic total coronary occlusions, it is imperative that one considers the clinical and coronary landscape (i.e. what is the risk of perforation or damage to collateral vessels) when considering what equipment is likely to be required to achieve procedural success. Coronary CTOs that are most likely to be uncrossable can often be identified by review of the initial angiograms. Many of these criteria remain unchanged from the original descriptive studies by Stone and others.[14,15,16-18] These criteria that predict failure by standard wire-based techniques (dense calcification, long occluded segments, lesions on bends, etc.) often reflect technical challenges for catheter-based laser systems as well. The prior literature reviewing recanalization of CTOs identified the duration of occlusion and attempts after prior CABG as the clinically important predictors of failure. The angiographic findings predictive of failure include the lesion morphology, especially the degree of calcification, length of the missing segment, presence of bridging collaterals, side branches at the site of occlusion, presence of significant angulation greater than 45°, and multilesion occlusions.

The current literature suggests that the failure rate for attempting CTO angioplasty still occurs in 15–50% of procedures.[19-22] Failure to cross the lesion with a primary wire and failure to cross the lesions with a therapeutic device are two important limitations in successfully treating CTOs. Preprocedure evaluation before attempting a CTO with one of the above clinical or angiographic predictors should include a specific decision about what procedures will be attempted if standard wires will not cross the lesion. Excimer laser atherectomy is appealing in this situation, as it provides an active ablative energy source that can ablate thrombus, collagen, and calcium. Laser catheters have been utilized to treat CTO since the introduction of the technology in the late 1980s.[23-29] Studies involving the excimer laser and the holmium[30] laser, the two systems evaluated in CTO and uncrossable lesions, are listed in Table 16.1. These registry studies demonstrate that device success has improved with the introduction of new techniques and catheter systems. As mentioned above, the holmium laser system is no longer available for clinical use. Improvements in the technique of laser atherectomy have also been significant in improving outcomes. The use of saline infusion during laser therapy removes the contrast media and red blood cells that decrease the photoacoustic effect.[31-34] This technical change has decreased the incidence of major dissections at the treatment site. During the treatment of uncrossable lesions or CTOs with laser, we can use the photoacoustic effect to our advantage with small catheters to achieve larger more complaints lumens post procedure. Therefore, the need for saline flush, which is indicated during laser treatment of non-occlusive stenoses, is not warranted.

In the late 1990s a novel wire-based laser technology was also developed and tested in two randomized trials, the TOTAL trial and the US TOTAL trial.[35,36] While the Laser Wire was found to be safe in the randomized trials, it was not

Table 16.1　Studies of laser atherectomy for uncrossable lesions or chronic total occlusions[a]

	n	Device success (%)	In-hospital MACE (%)	Comments
ELCA				
Schofer	80	90	1.2	Minor dissection (45%); restenosis (53%, with a 20% reocclusion rate)
Klein	172 (>3 months) 107 (<3 months)	85 90	2.0	Acute closure (4.5% vs 2.7%); perforation (0% vs 0.9%)
Baumbach[34]	212	–	–	Total occlusion predictive of perforation
Holme[29]	172	90	3.7	
Bittl[23]	127	84	–	
Holmium laser				
de Marchena (1994)	25	100	0	

[a]The series are relatively small but with high success rates. The in-hospital MACE rate is acceptably low. ELCA, excimer laser coronary angioplasty; MACE, major adverse cardiac events.

more effective than balloon catheter procedures alone. The most frequent reason for failure was still the inability to cross the lesion with the wire rather than failure of the laser device to cross the lesion. The prolonged procedure time and the failure to demonstrate improvement in procedural success contravened further development of this concept.

Recently, the excimer laser has undergone further improvements with much smaller profile catheters (0.9 and 0.7 mm), optimized laser fiber distribution for greater energy delivery, and continuous delivery of laser energy. Figure 16.2 demonstrates the difference in technique and improved ablative efficiency in an ex-vivo model comparing the 1.4 mm catheter with the 0.9 mm catheter. These changes have significantly improved the ability of the excimer laser to cross more complex lesions. This system, by virtue of increased laser energy delivered to the lesion, is also more facile in crossing long and calcified lesions than any previous device. Bilodeau et al,[37] have evaluated the use of the new 0.9 mm laser catheter to facilitate treatment of complex, calcified, and uncrossable lesions. This system improved technical success to 92% and clinical success to 86% in patients with lesions deemed not treatable using conventional balloon therapy. As we approach a larger number of patients with increasingly complex coronary lesions, the potential for application of excimer laser coronary atherectomy will increase. Additionally, the use of the same techniques will improve the operator's success when faced with an 'uncrossable lesion'. There are no contemporary randomized trials to help us understand the specific role of excimer laser vs other ablative technologies. Each physician will need to develop expertise with these devices to decide what role they might play in these complex lesion subsets. A representative case using laser to recanalize a CTO prior to stent placement is seen in Figure 16.3.

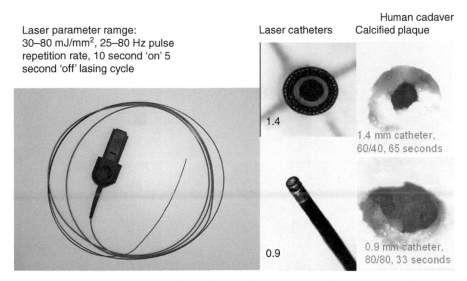

Figure 16.2 Laser catheter comparison: a 1.4 mm laser catheter and a 0.9 mm laser catheter. The smaller catheter has a more effective spacing of fibers as well as delivering more energy. The panel on the left demonstrates the increased effectiveness of the 0.9 mm catheter.

In-stent stenosis represents an additional lesion subset that is difficult to treat and may include long total occlusions. Many of the lesions in stent are formed from a long fibrous lesion that is difficult to cross with standard wire techniques and is not amenable to extravascular wire passage. The laser catheter is an excellent adjunct to recanalize these lesions.[38-40]

CHRONIC TOTAL OCCLUSIONS OF PERIPHERAL VESSELS

The need for peripheral artery revascularization is frequently seen in patients who have complex coronary artery disease. While revascularization of TASC 1 lesions has a high success rate and a high primary patency rate, these lesions are patent, short, non-angulated, and not severely calcified. The patients at greatest risk of severe peripheral disease are those patients with concomitant coronary artery disease and those who have multilevel obstruction.[41-43] Multilevel obstruction is often associated with long, calcified lesions of the superficial femoral artery, infrapopliteal disease, and/or chronic limb ischemia. Currently, these lesions are not recommended for revascularization based upon the ACC/AHA (American College of Cardiology/American Heart Association) guidelines published in 2005.[44] These long lesions have a lower procedural success rate and a greater likelihood of requiring a second procedure. One advantage of the laser catheter has been the decreased number and size of embolic particles seen after in-vitro and in-vivo laser atherectomy procedures. This allows the operator to have greater confidence in proceeding on to complete the entire procedure in a single setting.

Over the last 10 years, we have learned many important lessons about the technique for performing peripheral laser atherectomy. Many of these lessons

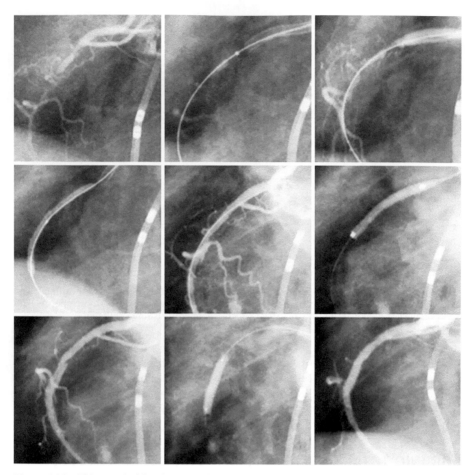

Figure 16.3   This panel of fixed images demonstrates the use of a 0.9 mm laser catheter to cross a totally occluded right coronary artery (RCA). After laser atherectomy, the lesion is ballooned and in the lower panels a stent is placed in the mid RCA.

are the same as those discussed above in approaching complex coronary lesions. The technique of advancement has undergone the most change. It is currently recommended that the operator advance the laser in a contrast-free environment at a very slow rate (<1 mm/s). If possible, one should also use a saline flush, starting just prior to initiating the laser energy and continuing during the entire laser pulse delivery. As noted above, the excimer laser is very effective at disrupting thrombus, even at a distance from the laser tip. This feature is very important when approaching long lesions or small-vessel disease, both of which are more likely to contain thrombus. Larger catheters and balloons may 'bulldoze' thrombus distally as the catheter is advanced. This can occlude side branches or result in distal occlusion during the procedure, requiring alternate devices or pharmacological therapy. Laser atherectomy is also useful for treatment of in-stent restenosis.

In long total occlusions, a new technique of advancing the catheter and wire independently is being utilized. This technique dubbed the 'step by step' technique is shown in Figure 16.4. This method departs from standard teaching and the technique for coronary procedures. The laser catheter is initially advanced over the wire into the lesion. Next, the laser catheter is activated and advanced several millimeters. When the laser catheter is deactivated, the wire is then readvanced ahead of the laser catheter and the procedure repeated until the entire totally occluded segment has been crossed. One can then use a larger laser catheter, balloon, or stent as clinically indicated. This technique is felt to produce a 'smoother' lumen than balloon angioplasty. If true, this might improve acute and long-term outcomes. These long complex lesions are typically fibrotic and are easily treated with excimer laser atherectomy. A typical picture of the baseline image and the postprocedure angiogram is seen in Figure 16.5. In calcified lesions, the laser catheter is often set at a higher fluence (energy setting) and more frequent pulses to increase the total amount of energy delivered to the lesion. This aggressive approach to peripheral vessel angioplasty is accompanied by a slightly higher rate of perforations, but these are easily treated with low-pressure occlusive balloon dilatation. The trade off is that one uses fewer stents in the peripheral arteries using excimer laser atherectomy. Clinical trials and registries of excimer laser for peripheral artery disease have been reported in several formats. Scheinert et al[45] reviewed their experience with 318 consecutive patients

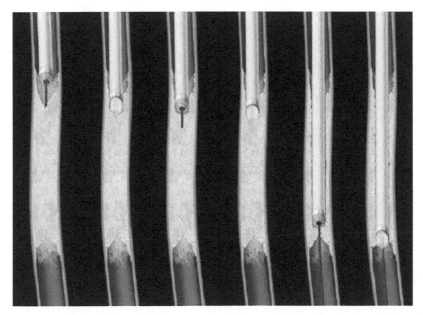

Figure 16.4 Peripheral laser atherectomy, referred to as the 'Step by Step' technique. The laser is advanced over the wire until resistance is felt. The laser catheter is then activated, and advanced several millimeters while the laser is activated. The wire is then readvanced until resistance is met and the procedure repeated until the catheter passes into the distal vessel lumen.

(a)

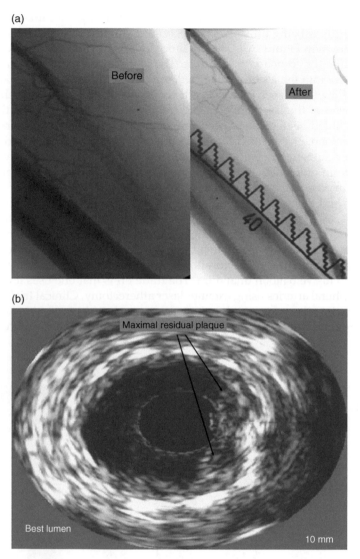

(b)

Figure 16.5 A case of in-stent stenosis within a superficial femoral artery (SFA) stent. The neointimal hyperplasia is ablated using an eccentric laser catheter with restoration of an excellent lumen and minimal residual neointima by intravascular ultrasound (IVUS) examination. (Courtesy of Craig Walker MD.)

(mean age 64 ± 10.7 years) with 411 lesions who underwent excimer laser-assisted revascularization with long lesions (19.4 ± 6.0 cm). The technical success rate was very high at 372 of 411 (90.5%). This investigation sparked interest in the concept of laser-assisted peripheral angioplasty and was followed by several other investigations.

The Peripheral Excimer Laser Angioplasty (PELA) trial[46] study was a multicenter, prospective, randomized trial comparing excimer laser-assisted percutaneous transluminal angioplasty (PTA) vs PTA. The investigation evaluated 251 patients with Rutherford category 2–4 for >6 months' duration and total occlusions ≥10 cm in the superticial femoral artery (SFA) were randomized (50% laser + PTA, 50% PTA alone) at 13 US sites and six German sites. Stenting was optional but discouraged. Clinical success was defined as primary patency (≤50% diameter stenosis at 1 year by ultrasound without reintervention) and absence of serious adverse events (SAE) defined as death, MI, vascular surgical repair, amputation, bypass, and acute limb ischemia. Acute procedural results from a preliminary analysis.

Follow-up reported from 189 PELA study patients was similar in both laser and balloon groups. Procedural success was lower, at 85% in the laser group and 91% in the PTA group. Total procedural complications were 12.8% and 11.4%, respectively. The only significant difference between the two groups was in the number of stents (42% laser vs 59% PTA) with similar 12-month patency.

The most complex patient subset is chronic limb ischemia. This subset of patients typically have more comorbid conditions and are the most likely to have limb amputation as the only alternative strategy.[47-49] The use of excimer laser atherectomy has been tested in this population in two trial settings.[50] The Laser Angioplasty for Critical Limb Ischemia (LACI) Phase 2[51-53] was designed to prospectively evaluate Rutherford class 4–6 patients who were poor bypass candidates with SFA, popliteal, or infrapopliteal vessels: 145 patients with 155 critically ischemic limbs and 433 lesions were enrolled in the trial. This high-risk patient population is significant for the presence of diabetes in 66% of patients and hypertension in 87%. Ischemia had been present for 25 ± 37 weeks, reflecting the chronicity of this process. In this subset, 70% of patients had combinations of stenosis and occlusions at multiple levels. Table reviews the results of this interesting trial. The guidewire passage failed in 8% but was recovered by using the step by step technique to advance the laser across the lesions. Ultimately, 99% of lesions were crossed and a balloon was delivered to 94% of the lesions. The clinically important measure of success is the achievement of straight line flow in the lower extremity. In the LACI trial, 89% of patients had restoration of this flow. Despite the complexity of these patients, they only remained in the hospital an average of 3 days.

The clinical outcomes after revascularization are thought provoking in this very high-risk patient group. SAE during the 6-month enrollment period included 10% mortality, predominately from cardiac causes. Major amputation was required in 11 cases, whereas four limbs received surgical reintervention. An additional 24 limbs required endovascular reinterventions to reopen lesions. At 6-month follow-up, limb salvage was achieved in 118 of 127 (93%) limbs. Representative pictures are seen in Figures 16.6 and 16.7. While population studies are important, these individual findings serve to demonstrate what can be achieved in some high-risk patients who are not candidates for surgical revascularization.

CONCLUSIONS

The catheters and technique for performing laser atherectomy have significantly improved since its introduction in the late 1980s. The development of smaller

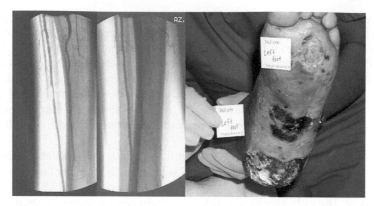

Figure 16.6 Images from a peripheral angioplasty in a patient with chronic limb ischemia. This is not a chronically occluded vessel but might be difficult to treat using standard balloon angioplasty. The middle panel demonstrates the result post laser therapy. (Courtesy of John Laird MD.)

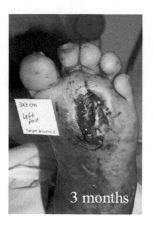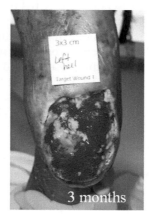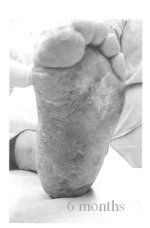

Figure 16.7 The panels demonstrate the healing that occurred in the patient from Figure 16.6 after restoration of blood flow. (Courtesy of John Laird MD.)

more powerful lasers, delivering continuous energy, facilitates the ablative atherectomy required for treating longer more complex lesions and chronically occluded vessels. Understanding the mechanisms of laser ablation and following the procedural guidelines that minimize the photoacoustic effect by infusing saline and slowly advancing the catheter will optimize procedural outcomes.

Aggressive treatment of chronically occluded coronary arteries improves the operator's ability to restore antegrade flow, improving patients' long-term outcomes. Whereas a laser is likely to be required in only a small percentage of CTOs, using a laser is likely to improve the procedural success and to decrease the time required to accomplish these procedures. Extension of this technique to the more frequent problems of the difficult-to-cross or uncrossable lesion will simplify the procedure and allow operators to maintain their skill in performing the procedure.

Peripheral angioplasty has more opportunity for the use of excimer laser atherectomy as an integral part of the procedure. While TASC 1 lesions are approved as class I indications for endovascular revascularization, the majority of patients currently being evaluated have longer, more complex lesions which are often chronically occluded and present at multiple levels. The use of a laser as part of this strategy will increase the number of lesions that can be treated and hopefully further improve late outcomes.

REFERENCES

1. Srivasta SS, Edwards WE, Boos CM, et al. Histologic correlates of angiographic chronic total coronary artery occlusions: influence of occlusion duration on neovascular channel patterns and intimal plaque composition. J Am Coll Cardiol 1997; 29:955–63.
2. Katsuragawa M, Fujiwara H, Miyamae M, et al. Histologic studies in percutaneous transluminal coronary angioplasty for chronic total occlusions: comparison of tapering and abrupt types of occlusion and short and long occluded segments. J Am Coll Cardiol 1993; 21: 604–11.
3. Aziz S, Ramsdale DR. Chronic total occlusions – a stiff challenge requiring a major breakthrough: is there light at the end of the tunnel? Heart 2005; 91(Suppl3):iii42–8.
4. Isner JM, Rosenfield K, White CJ, et al. In vivo assessment of vascular pathology resulting from laser irradiation. Analysis of 23 patients studied by directional atherectomy immediately after laser angioplasty Circulation 1992; 85:2185–96.
5. Bonner R, Smith P, Prevosti L, et al. New sources for laser angioplasty: Er:YAG, excimer lasers, and nonlaser hot-tip catheters. In:Vogel J, King S, eds. Interventional Cardiology: Future Directions. St Louis: Mosby; 1989:101–8.
6. Korovin N. Spectral differences between normal and atherosclerotic aorta. Magill J Med 1999; 5:5–12.
7. Clarke RH, Isner JM, Donaldson RF, Jones G 2nd. Gas chromatographic-light microscopic correlative analysis of excimer laser photoablation of cardiovascular tissues: evidence for a thermal mechanism. Circ Res 1987; 60:429–37.
8. Litvack F, Forrester J, Grundfest W, et al. The excimer laser: from basic science to clinical application. In: Vogel J, King SB, eds. Interventional Cardiology: Future Directions. St Louis: Mosby; 1989:170–81.
9. Lee G, Ikeda RM, Stobbe D, et al. Effects of laser irradiation on human thrombus: demonstration of a linear dissolution-dose relation between clot length and energy density. Am J Cardiol 1983; 52;876–7.
10. Topaz O, Minisi A, Bernardo NL, et al. Alterations of platelet aggregation kinetics with ultraviolet laser emission: the "stunned platelet" phenomenon. Thromb Haemost 2001; 86:1087–93.
11. Dahm JB, Topaz O, Woenckhaus C, et al. Laser-facilitated thrombectomy: a new therapeutic option for treatment of thrombus-laden coronary lesions. Catheter Cardiovasc Interv 2002; 56(3):365–72.
12. Shangguan HQ, Gregory KW, Casperson LW, Prahl SA. Enhanced laser thrombolysis with photomechanical drug delivery: an in vitro study. Lasers Surg Med 1998; 23:151–60.
13. Olivari Z, Rubartelli P, Piscione F, et al. TOAST-GISE Investigators. Immediate results and one-year clinical outcome after percutaneous coronary interventions in chronic total occlusions: data from a multicenter, prospective, observational study (TOAST-GISE). J Am Coll Cardiol 2003; 41(10):1672–8.
14. Stone GW, Rutherford BD, McConahay DR, et al. Procedural outcome of angioplasty for total coronary artery occlusion: an analysis of 971 lesions in 905 patients. J Am Coll Cardiol 1990; 15:849–56.

15. Stone GW, Rutherford BD, McConahay DR, et al. Procedural outcome of angioplasty for total coronary artery occlusion: an analysis of 971 lesions in 905 patients. J Am Coll Cardiol 1990; 15:849–56.
16. Dong S, Smorgick Y, Nadir M, et al. Predictors for successful angioplasty of chronic totally occluded coronary arteries. J Interv Cardiol 2005; 18:1–7.
17. Betge S, Krack A, Figulla HR, Werner GS. Analysis of location and pattern of target vessel failure in chronic total occlusions after stent implantation and its potential for the efficient use of drug-eluting stents. J Interv Cardiol 2006; 19(3):226–31.
18. Fang CC, Jao YT, Chen Y, Wang SP. Coronary stenting or balloon angioplasty for chronic total coronary occlusions: the Taiwan experience (a single-center report). Angiology 2005; 56(5):525–37.
19. Ivanhoe RJ, Weintraub WS, Douglas JS Jr, et al. Percutaneous transluminal coronary angioplasty of chronic total occlusions. Primary success, restenosis and long term clinical follow-up. Circulation 1992; 85:106–15.
20. Angioi M, Danchin N, Juilliere Y, et al., Is percutaneous transluminal coronary angioplasty in chronic total coronary occlusion justified? Long term results in a series of 201 patients. Arch Mal Coeur Vaiss 1995; 88:1383–9.
21. Noguchi T, Miyazaki S, Morii I, et al. Percutaneous transluminal coronary angioplasty of chronic total occlusions. Determinants of primary success and long-term clinical outcome. Catheter Cardiovasc Interv 2000; 49:258–64.
22. Suero JA, Marso SP, Jones PG, et al. Procedural outcomes and long-term survival among patients undergoing percutaneous coronary intervention of a chronic total occlusion in native coronary arteries: a 20-year experience. J Am Coll Cardiol 2001; 38:409–14.
23. Bittl JA, Sanborn TA, Tcheng JE, et al. Clinical success, complications and restenosis rates with excimer laser coronary angioplasty. The Percutaneous Excimer Laser Coronary Angioplasty Registry. Am J Cardiol 1992; 70:1533–9.
24. Litvack F, Eigler N, Margolis J, et al. Percutaneous excimer laser coronary angioplasty: results in the first consecutive 3,000 patients. The ELCA Investigators. J Am Coll Cardiol 1994; 23:323–9.
25. Appelman Y, Koolen J, Piek J, et al. Excimer laser angioplasty versus balloon angioplasty in functional and total coronary occlusions. Am J Cardiol 1996; 78:757–62.
26. Litvack F, Eigler N, Margolis J, et al. Percutaneous excimer laser coronary angioplasty: Results in the first consecutive 3,000 patients. The ELCA Investigators. J Am Coll Cardiol 1994; 23:323–9.
27. Appelman YE, Piek JJ, Strikwerda S, et al. Randomised trial of excimer laser angioplasty versus balloon angioplasty for treatment of obstructive coronary artery disease. Lancet 1996; 347:79–84.
28. Appelman YE, Piek JJ, Redekop WK, et al. Clinical events following excimer laser angioplasty or balloon angioplasty for complex coronary lesions: subanalysis of a randomised trial. Heart 1998; 79:34–8.
29. Holmes DR, Mehta S, George CJ, et al. Excimer laser coronary angioplasty: the New Approaches to Coronary Intervention (NACI) experience. Am J Cardiol 1997; 80:99–105K.
30. Stone GW, de Marchena E, Dageforde D, et al. Prospective, randomized, multicenter comparison of laser-facilitated balloon angioplasty versus stand-alone balloon angioplasty in patients with obstructive coronary artery disease. The Laser Angioplasty Versus Angioplasty (LAVA) Trial Investigators. J Am Coll Cardiol 1997; 30:1714–21.
31. Isner J, Pickering J, Mosseri M. Laser-induced dissections: pathogenesis and implications for therapy. J Am Coll Cardiol 1992; 19:1619–21.
32. Tcheng JE, Wells LD, Phillips HR, et al. Development of a new technique for reducing pressure pulse generation during 308-nm excimer laser coronary angioplasty. Cathet Cardiovasc Diagn 1995; 34:15–22.
33. Deckelbaum LI, Natarajan MK, Bittl JA, et al. Effect of intracoronary saline infusion on dissection during excimer laser coronary angioplasty: a randomized trial. The Percutaneous Excimer Laser Coronary Angioplasty (PELCA) Investigators. J Am Coll Cardiol 1995; 26:1264–9.

34. Baumbach A, Bittl JA, Fleck E, et al. Acute complications of excimer laser coronary angioplasty: a detailed analysis of multicenter results. Coinvestigators of the U.S. and European Percutaneous Excimer Laser Coronary Angioplasty (PELCA) Registries. J Am Coll Cardiol 1994; 23:1305–13.
35. Oesterle SN, Bittl JA, Leon MB, et al. Laser wire for crossing chronic total occlusions: "learning phase" results from the U.S. TOTAL trial. Total Occlusion Trial With Angioplasty by Using a Laser Wire. Cathet Cardiovasc Diagn 1998; 44:235–43.
36. Serruys PW, Hamburger J, Koolen JJ, et al. Total occlusion trial with angioplasty by using laser guidewire. The TOTAL trial. Eur Heart J 2000; 21:1797–805.
37. Bilodeau L, Fretz EB, Taeymans Y, et al. Novel use of a high-energy excimer laser catheter for calcified and complex coronary artery lesions. Catheter Cardiovasc Interv 2004; 62:155–61.
38. Bittl JA, Kuntz RE, Estella P, et al. Analysis of late lumen narrowing after excimer laser-facilitated coronary angioplasty. J Am Coll Cardiol 1994; 23:1314–20.
39. Koster R, Hamm CW, Terres W, et al. Treatment of in-stent coronary restenosis by excimer laser angioplasty. Am J Cardiol 1997; 80:1424–8.
40. Mehran R, Mintz GS, Satler LF, et al. Treatment of in-stent restenosis with excimer laser coronary angioplasty: mechanisms and results compared with PTCA alone. Circulation 1997; 96:2183–9.
41. Criqui MH, Denenberg JO, Langer RD, Fronek A. The epidemiology of peripheral arterial disease: importance of identifying the population at risk. Vasc Med 1997; 2:221–6.
42. Ness J, Aronow WS. Prevalence of coexistence of coronary artery disease, ischemic stroke, and peripheral arterial disease in older persons, mean age 80 years, in an academic hospital-based geriatrics practice. J Am Geriatr Soc 1999; 47:1255– 6.
43. Biamino G. The excimer laser: science fiction fantasy or practical tool? J Endovasc Ther 2004; 11(Suppl 2):ii207–22.
44. Hirsch AT, Haskal ZJ, Hertzer NR, et al. ACC/AHA 2005 Practice Guidelines for the management of patients with peripheral arterial disease (lower extremity, renal, mesenteric and abdominal aortic). Circulation 2006; 113:e463–654.
45. Scheinert D, Laird JR Jr, Schroder M, et al. Excimer laser-assisted recanalization of long, chronic superficial femoral artery occlusions. J Endovasc Ther 2001; 8:156–66.
46. Laird JR Jr, Reiser C, Biamino G, Zeller T. Excimer laser assisted angioplasty for the treatment of critical limb ischemia. J Cardiovasc Surg (Torino) 2004; 45:239–48.
47. Bosiers M, Peeters P, Elst FV, et al. Excimer laser assisted angioplasty for critical limb ischemia: results of the LACI Belgium Study. Eur J Vasc Endovasc Surg 2005; 29:613–19.
48. Gray BH, Laird JR, Ansel GM, Shuck JW. Complex endovascular treatment for critical limb ischemia in poor surgical candidates: a pilot study. J Endovasc Ther 2002; 9:599–604.
49. Weitz JI, Byrne J, Clagett GP, et al. Diagnosis and treatment of chronic arterial insufficiency of the lower extremities: a critical review. Circulation 1996; 94:3026–49.
50. Biamino G, Scheinert D. Excimer laser treatment of SFA occlusions. Endovasc Today 2003:May/June.
51. Laird JR. Laser Angioplasty for Critical Limb Ischemia (LACI): results of the LACI Phase 2 Clinical Trial. Presented at ISET Annual Meeting, January 2003.
52. Laird JR. Laser Angioplasty for Critical Limb Ischemia (LACI): results of the LACI Phase 2 Clinical Trial. Presented at ISET Annual Meeting, January 2003.
53. Laird JR, Zeller T, Gray B, et al. Limb salvage following laser-assisted angioplasty for critical limb ischemia: results of the LACI multicenter trial. J Endovasc Ther 2006; 13:1–11.

17

Role of antegrade blunt dissection for coronary and peripheral chronic total occlusions

Patrick L Whitlow and Matthew Selmon

Coronary Frontrunner experience • Peripheral artery experience with the Frontrunner and Outback LTD reentry catheter • Conclusions

The Frontrunner catheter was originally designed to open chronic total occlusions (CTOs) of coronary and peripheral arteries refractory to guidewire recanalization. The device works by creating blunt microdissection, taking advantage of the increased elastic properties of the arterial wall compared with plaque. When pressure is applied, adventitia stretches to a far greater degree than atherosclerotic plaque; therefore, when adequate force is applied, plaque will separate while the arterial wall stretches, theoretically opening a channel through the occlusion that can then be recanalized with a guidewire, balloon, and stenting techniques. Differential elasticity permits the plaque to be separated without causing arterial perforation (Figure 17.1).

CORONARY FRONTRUNNER EXPERIENCE

The original Frontrunner device for coronary artery application was 4.5 Fr in size (Figure 17.2). This size mandated utilization of an 8 Fr guiding catheter for contrast injections in order to safely guide Frontrunner advancement through the artery to the occlusion. In the original multicenter registry of the Frontrunner for coronary artery CTOs, 107 patients failing guidewire techniques for at least 10 minutes of fluoroscopy time were entered into the trial. The mean lesion length in the registry was 22 mm, with a range of 2–53 mm. The Frontrunner was successfully delivered to the CTO in 89.7% of cases. The device was passed into the lesion and a wire was placed into the distal true lumen of the artery in 56.1% of cases.

Complications included two Frontrunner perforations (1.9%), which were asymptomatic and caused no hemodynamic compromise. These cases were treated by withdrawing the Frontrunner and reversing the heparin. Additionally,

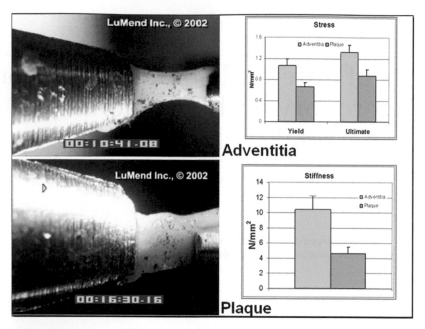

Figure 17.1   Comparison of CTO tissues (adventitia and fibrous plaque).

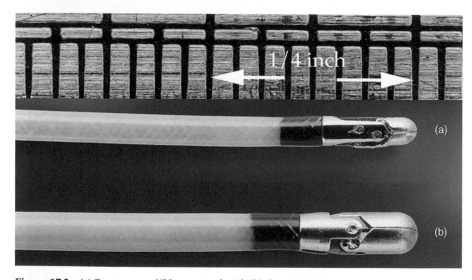

Figure 17.2   (a) Frontrunner X39 compared with (b) the original Frontrunner.

there were three guidewire perforations and one stent perforation. In these four cases, two patients were treated with pericardiocentesis for impending tamponade. No surgical intervention was required.[1]

In this registry, proximal right coronary occlusions had the lowest success rate of any other anatomical location (Table 17.1). This was felt to be due to the

Table 17.1   Frontrunner success by lesion location

	Left circumflex	LAD	RCA
Proximal	70%	64%	44%
Mid-distal	56%	50%	71%
Overall	63%	57%	54%

LAD, left anterior descending coronary artery; RCA, right coronary artery.

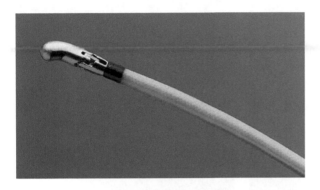

Figure 17.3   Frontrunner with a curved tip (Frontrunner XR).

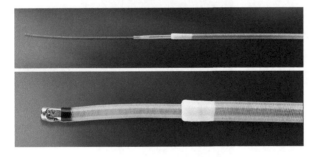

Figure 17.4   Frontrunner Micro Guide Catheter is shown first with the obturator and second with the Frontrunner preloaded.

Frontrunner catheter migrating to the outer edge of the major curve of the proximal right coronary artery (RCA). Therefore, a Frontrunner catheter with a curved distal tip was designed (Figure 17.3). The curve was meant to enable the operator to steer the device more to the inner aspect of the RCA proximal curve. However, success in the proximal RCA was never equal to other locations.

Further iterations of the Frontrunner included downsizing the device to 0.039 inch (2.8 Fr) and making the distal curve retention of the instrument more robust. The Frontrunner X39 in a straight version became the preferred Frontrunner catheter in 2004 (see Figure 17.2a). This catheter could be utilized in a 6 Fr guide. The reduced shaft size also allowed combination with a microguide catheter (Figure 17.4), which allowed replacement of the Frontrunner with a guidewire once the lesion was crossed or at the operator's discretion. The adjunctive use of the microguide catheter requires a 7 Fr guiding catheter.

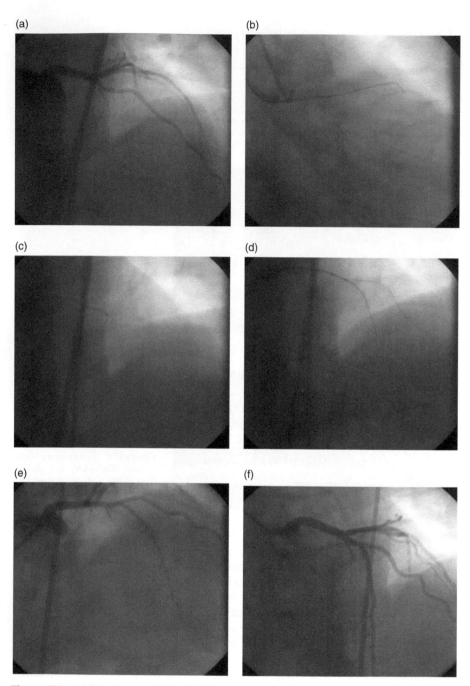

Figure 17.5 (a) Simultaneous left and right coronary injections showing a long mid LAD (left anterior descending coronary artery) occlusion that is 12 years old. (b) Parallel guidewires were unsuccessful in entering the distal true lumen. (c) The Frontrunner is used to penetrate the proximal fibrous cap. (d) A Miraclebros 3 wire is used to cross the chronic total occlusion (CTO). (e) Final results after a drug-eluting stent is placed. (f) Six month follow-up showing continued success of the CTO.

Orlic et al published their results of using the Frontrunner for extremely challenging patients in 2005.[2] Of the 50 consecutive CTO patients, 32 failed conventional wire techniques and 18 were felt 'unsuitable' for conventional techniques because of difficult anatomy. The occlusion length averaged 38 ± 22 mm and 72% of the lesions were at least 20 mm in length. After using the Frontrunner, a guidewire could subsequently be passed successfully into the distal true lumen in 50% of the cases. In 68% of these successful cases, the Frontrunner alone could enter into the distal true lumen without adjunctive use of a wire and in 32% the Frontrunner was used to cross the initial fibrous cap and a wire was used to cross the remainder of the CTO. The 50% success rate in refractory cases was associated with a significant complication rate, however. Overall, the incidence of perforation was 14%. There was a significant decrease in the incidence of perforation from cases in year 1 to year 2, from 41.7% to 10.5%, indicating a learning curve for the device. Pericardiocentesis was required in two (4%) patients.

With improvements in wire technology and technique, the Frontrunner has emerged as a tool for refractory CTO cases failing new guidewire technology. Case 1 (Figure 17.5) is an example of a man with a 12-year-old occlusion of the mid-LAD (left anterior descending coronary artery) that failed aggressive guidewire attempts. Guidewire attempts were abandoned and the proximal fibrous cap was then re-crossed with the Frontrunner. This new entry enabled an Asahi Miraclebros 3 wire to traverse the lesion in the true lumen. This wire was successfully steered into the distal LAD and the LAD was then recanalized with a Cypher stent. Follow-up catheterization 6 months later documented wide patency from this CTO intervention.

PERIPHERAL ARTERY EXPERIENCE WITH THE FRONTRUNNER AND OUTBACK LTD REENTRY CATHETER

A new Frontrunner platform was developed for use in CTOs of peripheral arteries. The Frontrunner XP Peripheral CTO Catheter is 0.039 inch (2.8 Fr) distal tip size (Figure 17.6). The catheter comes in 90 and 140 cm working length sizes.

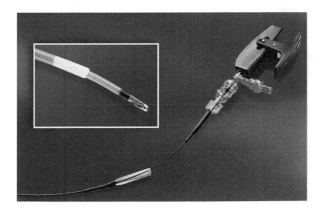

Figure 17.6 The Frontrunner XP Catheter is 0.039 inch in diameter and designed specifically for peripheral application.

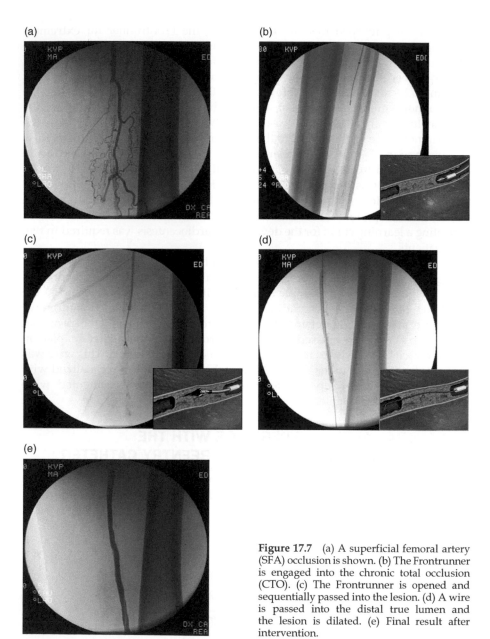

Figure 17.7   (a) A superficial femoral artery (SFA) occlusion is shown. (b) The Frontrunner is engaged into the chronic total occlusion (CTO). (c) The Frontrunner is opened and sequentially passed into the lesion. (d) A wire is passed into the distal true lumen and the lesion is dilated. (e) Final result after intervention.

The XP has a more robust distal tip for improved lesion engagement and tip shapeability with an 0.008 inch pull wire for more forceful jaw opening and tip shape retention. The device also has greater shaft flexibility for improved distal torque control, going around the aortic bifurcation and down the contralateral leg. For a contralateral superficial femoral artery (SFA) occlusion, a crossover sheath is placed; then, the Frontrunner Micro Guide Catheter is placed over

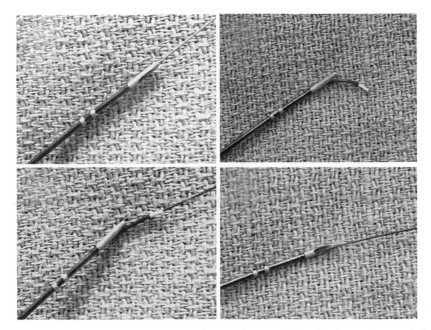

Figure 17.8   The Outback LTD Reentry Catheter is shown with the distal cannula extended.

an 0.35 inch wire near the proximal CTO. The Frontrunner catheter is then inserted and engaged using a road-mapped image. The catheter is advanced into the CTO and the jaws are opened. Then, the catheter is closed and pulled back slightly to make sure that there is no tissue trapped in the tip. The catheter is then rotated slightly and engaged further and reopened. This sequence is repeated until the CTO is crossed or until the operator decides to change out for a guidewire attempt (Figure 17.7). If the distal true lumen cannot be entered, frequently a subintimal position next to the distal true lumen can be visualized. If this occurs, the Outback LTD catheter can be utilized for true lumen reentry (Figure 17.8).

The Outback LTD catheter utilizes a sharp nitinol cannula that can be extended from the end of the Outback into the distal true lumen for reentry. Through this hollow cannula, a 0.014 inch wire can be placed in the distal true lumen. The Outback LTD catheter can then be withdrawn and a balloon catheter passed over the 0.014 inch wire. The combination of the Frontrunner and Outback LTD catheter for reentry is very quick compared with guidewire manipulation in a long SFA total occlusion. An Outback LTD case is shown in Figure 17.9.

The Frontrunner catheter was acquired from LuMend, Inc., by Cordis Corporation (a Johnson & Johnson company) in early 2006. The company decided to suspend marketing the coronary Frontrunner X39 catheter indefinitely. However, the Frontrunner XP Peripheral Catheter and Outback LTD Reentry Catheter are still available for use.

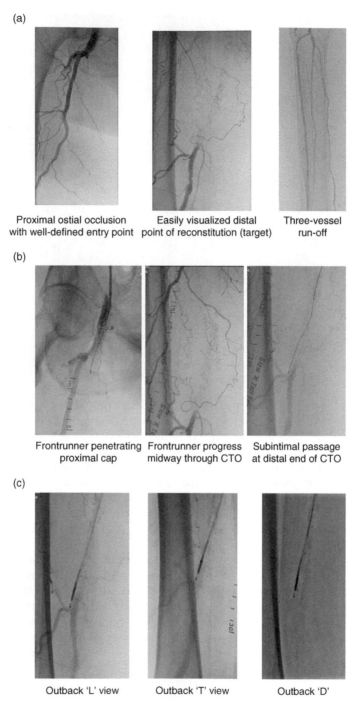

Figure 17.9 (Continued)

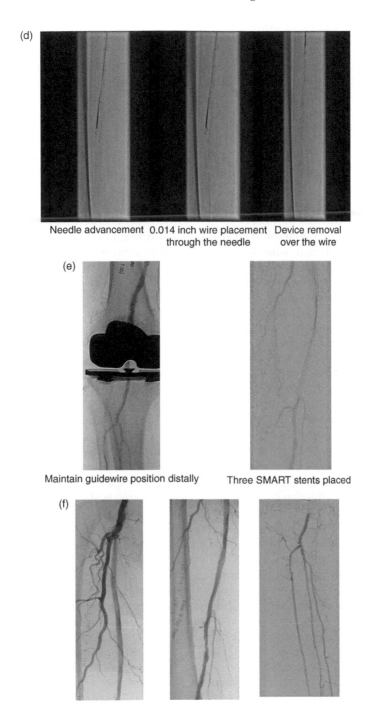

Figure 17.9 (Continued)

A 75-year-old male, with lifestyle-limiting claudication, and long right super-ficial femoral artery chronic total occlusion (SFA CTO). The ankle–brachial index (ABI) is 0.6 (Figure 17.9). The procedure steps are described concisely. (a) A long SFA CTO with diffuse proximal subtotal occlusion with disease involving the ostium of the profunda, and a mid-SFA complete occlusion of 15 cm with recon-stitution near Hunter's canal. The distal reconstitution pattern is very important and should be evaluated with angiography to delineate collaterals and vessel size in determining revascularization strategies. There is three-vessel run-off, which is an important determinant of favorable revascularization outcome. (b) Using a crossover sheath from the contralateral left femoral, the right SFA was entered with a Frontrunner catheter (FR) loaded into a Micro Guide Catheter (MGC). A small curve was placed on the distal end of the FR for steering, and then advanced through the area of subtotal occlusion. A blunt controlled microdissec-tion technique was used to advance the FR through the CTO to the distal area of SFA reconstitution. After the FR was advanced beyond the end of the CTO in a subintimal location, adjacent to the true distal lumen, repeated attempts to 'reenter' the true lumen with a guidewire were unsuccessful. (c) The Outback LTD catheter was then advanced in the most distal subintimal location as fol-lows: the MGC was advanced to the area of reconstitution over the FR, and then the FR was removed and an exchange length 0.014 inch guidewire was placed, and the MGC removed. An Outback LTD Reentry Catheter was then advanced over the 0.014 inch wire and positioned in the subintimal space adjacent to the reconstituted true lumen. The left image demonstrates the Outback LTD in the 'L' position with the distal 'L' marker pointing toward the true lumen. The image intensifier is positioned to maximize the perpendicular view of the catheter adja-cent to the true lumen. The image intensifier was then moved to a 90° orthogonal view, which shows the Outback superimposed on the adjacent true lumen, and the marker appears as a 'T.' The middle image demonstrates the 'T' configu-ration and shows the Outback superimposed on the distal true lumen. This view allows 'fine tuning' of the Outback position to maximize the direction of the reentry cannula. The cannula deployment 'D' step is shown in the right image. Once positioned in orthogonal views, the Outback cannula can be deployed in either view although it is best seen in the 'L' view. The Outback catheter was held firmly in position at the hub of the sheath to prevent the catheter from moving backwards during deployment of the cannula in the 'L' view. After the cannula is deployed, the guidewire is advanced into the true lumen and positioned distally in the vessel. (d) The steps of guidewire placement through the needle/cannula into the true lumen and into the distal vessel. Once the 0.014 inch guidewire is positioned distally, the cannula is retracted, and the Outback is removed over the guidewire. The reentry hole is then dilated with a balloon and allows antegrade blood flow. (e, left side) A distal injection after crossing back into the true lumen to confirm catheter position and distal anatomy. After the guidewire is posi-tioned distally in the true lumen, the case progresses with definitive therapy based on operator choice. This patient required stent implantation throughout the SFA lesion, yielding good in-line flow to the foot. (f) The final angiogram. The proximal vessel is imaged (left side) after stent implantation, but particular atten-tion is paid to the distal 'reentry' site (middle image) to confirm wide patency, and assure good run-off. The right side demonstrates angiography of the distal vessel following stent implantation, confirming a good angiographic result with brisk antegrade three-vessel run-off.

CONCLUSIONS

In summary, the Frontrunner X39 coronary catheter is a device useful to open approximately 50–60% of CTO cases refractory to guidewire techniques. However, this catheter is no longer available for clinical use. The Frontrunner XP for SFA/popliteal CTOs is currently available and often used with the Outback LTD Reentry Catheter. Ongoing registries are tracking utilization and success rates. Initial data look promising for utilizing these devices to cross long peripheral artery CTOs successfully and expediently with reduced fluoroscopy/procedure time compared with traditional guidewire techniques.

REFERENCES

1. Whitlow PL, Selmon M, O'Neill W, et al. Treatment of uncrossable chronic total coronary occlusions with the Frontrunner: multicenter experience. J Am Coll Cardiol 2002; 39 (Suppl 1): 29.
2. Orlic D, Stankovic G, Sangiorgi G, et al. Preliminary experience with the Frontrunner coronary catheter: novel device dedicated to mechanical revascularization of chronic total occlusions. Catheter Cardiovasc Interv 2005; 64(2):146–52..

18

Role of an optical reflectometry and radiofrequency ablation device: coronary chronic total occlusions

Gregory A Braden and George D Dangas

Case example • **Conclusion**

A special system aims to overcome the uncertainty of properly penetrating the proximal chronic total occlusion (CTO) cap vs exiting the vessel with the use of optical coherence reflectometry (OCR), and even contribute to fibrous cap weakening by a well-directed use of radiofrequency (RF) ablation.

The Safe-Cross RF guidewire (IntraLuminal Therapeutics, Carlsbad, CA) is an 0.014 inch intermediate-stiffness guidewire with the capacity to perform real-time OCR, and display the result in a dedicated monitor that can be viewed by the operator during wire manipulation (the device and monitor pictures are included in Chapter 20). The purpose of this feature is to notify the operator when the wire tip is about to exit the arterial wall.[1-3]

OCR assesses the reflection of near-infrared light from different distances ahead of the wire tip. Reflections from plaque and vessel wall differ according to the tissue structure and there is distinct secondary reflection peak from the organized structures in the media and adventitia. This should warn the operator at a distance of 1 mm from the outer arterial wall and allow redirection of the wire before vessel exit occurs. When proximity to the vessel wall is not detected, the Safe-Cross RF wire can also be used to deliver a short battery of RF energy pulses to the wire tip in order to modify the proximal CTO cap and facilitate wire passage through hard fibrotic material within the occluded segment.

Therefore, in addition to the navigation guidance and the ablation potential, this system should also be complemented with excellent wire-crossing properties. Owing to wire tip stiffness in the present system, it is mostly useful in straight CTO segments, or it may be used just to break up the fibrous cap and then be exchanged for another wire to continue advancement through the occlusion. The latter approach can be used at the beginning of the case, or after failure of conventional wires (in the absence of significant dissection plane).

After initial favorable pilot experiences conducted in selected centers,[1,2] the utility of this device was tested in the Guided Radio Frequency Energy Ablation of Total Occlusions (GREAT) Registry. This included 116 patients, enrolled in multiple sites and followed prospectively. A key inclusion criterion was the existence of a CTO refractory to a 10-minute attempt with conventional guidewires.[3] The median occlusion duration was 22 months, while 32% of CTO lesions were at least 1 year old. Median lesion length was 25 mm (range = 6–80 mm), whereas 25% of cases were longer then 30 mm. Unfavorable anatomical features were frequently present, such as bridging collaterals (54%) and blunt entry into the occluded segment (47%).

Device success, which was defined as achievement of guidewire position in the distal lumen, was achieved in 54% of cases and was independent of vessel location, occlusion duration, lesion morphology, and collateral type. Major adverse events occurred in 7% of patients, consisting mostly (5%) of postprocedural enzyme elevations; there were no procedure-related deaths, Q-wave myocardial infarctions, or emergency bypass operations. Clinically relevant perforations occurred in three patients (2.6% overall) without further complications; one was directly related to the Safe-Cross RF wire, and two occurred during use of guidewires used after the Safe-Cross RF had failed to cross the CTO length.

CASE EXAMPLE

This device was used to initiate the procedure of a distal right coronary CTO in a patient with persistent severe angina and normal left ventricular function (Figure 18.1). An 8 Fr AL1 guiding catheter was used, owing to moderate proximal and mid-vessel tortuosity before the occluded segment (Figure 18.1a); a conventional workhorse wire negotiated the distal coronary segment, followed by advancement of an end-hole support catheter. The wire was then exchanged for the straight Safe-Cross RF, since the occluded segment appeared short after a dual injection was performed. A mild bend was made in the end of the wire to facilitate manipulations. The OCR indicator verified the appropriate position of the wire, and RF ablation shots were delivered three times successfully.

Because this wire could not be advanced further and OCR indicated a position close to the vessel wall (Figure 18.1b), the wire was then exchanged for a Miraclebros 3 with a small bend at its tip. Severe tortuosity of the distal right coronary artery (RCA) segment was felt to limit the ability of this wire to penetrate further due to non-coaxial alignment with the main body of the occlusion. It was therefore left in place, the support catheter was removed, and reinserted over a conventional wire, which negotiated the proximal vessel and was exchanged to a Confianza Pro when it reached the CTO site. Following the parallel wire technique (Figure 18.1c, d; black arrow = initial wire, white arrow = crossing wire), during visualization of the occlusion in multiple projections, this wire was able to cross into the distal vessel (middle branch of the trifurcation, Figure 18.1e).

The appearance of the distal vessel included extensive dissection but brisk antegrade flow (Figure 18.1f) that improved with dilation with a 3.0/20 mm balloon at 12 atm for 3 minutes. The procedure was then terminated (Figure 18.1g, h); the pharmacological regimen included chronic use of aspirin and clopidogrel

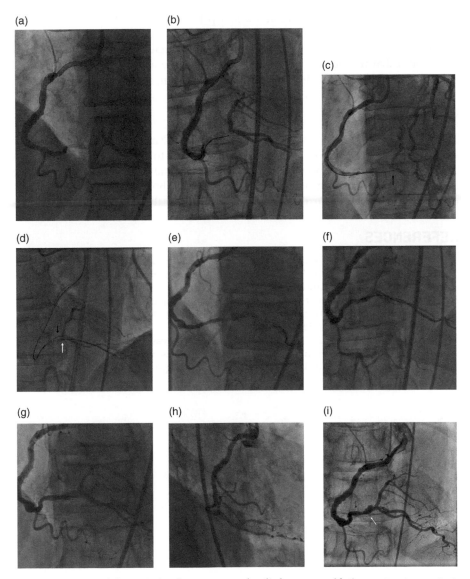

Figure 18.1 Use of the optical reflectometry and radiofrequency ablation system to penetrate the proximal cap of a coronary occlusion. The proceedure was completed with a non-hydrophilic guidewire. See text for step–by–step details.

(additional loading with 300 mg was performed) and heparin (3000 units at the beginning of the procedure and an additional 3000 units after wire cross, with activated clotting time [ACT] values of 205 to 295 seconds).

Complete resolution of symptoms was achieved and a 6-month follow-up angiogram indicated normal flow, a 25% residual stenosis, and healing of the dissection. Interestingly, it revealed a sharp bend (Figure 18.1i; from black to white arrows) within the previous occlusion that explained the inability of the Safe-Cross RF to succeed any further than the proximal fibrous cap. However, it is doubtful that the degree of tortuosity would have allowed adequate coaxial support for crossing of the lesion without special equipment.

CONCLUSION

This device can be an interesting addition to the CTO armamentarium as it provides unique features. An experienced operator has to choose when to use this device, how long to try, and when to convert to a classic CTO wire technique. The benefit of this specialty catheter may specifically be the initial penetration of the proximal cap, which in turn, can facilitate the use of other CTO wires.

REFERENCES

1. Cordero H, Warburton KD, Underwood PL, Heuser RR. Initial experience and safety in the treatment of chronic total occlusions with fiberoptic guidance technology: optical coherence reflectometry. Catheter Cardiovasc Interv 2001; 54:180–7.
2. Shammas NW. Treatment of chronic total occlusions using optical coherent reflectometry and radiofrequency ablative energy: incremental success over conventional techniques. J Invasive Cardiol 2004; 16:58–9.
3. Baim DS, Braden G, Heuser R, et al. Utility of the Safe-Cross-guided radiofrequency total occlusion crossing system in chronic coronary total occlusions (Results from the Guided Radio Frequency Energy Ablation of Total Occlusions Registry Study). Am J Cardiol 2004; 94:853–8.

19

Role of an optical reflectometry and radiofrequency ablation device: peripheral chronic total occlusions

M Ishti Ali and Richard Heuser

Introduction • ILT Safe-Cross RF system • Physics of optical coherence
reflectometry • GRIP trial • Case review • Conclusion

INTRODUCTION

Peripheral arterial disease affects 10 million people in the USA, approximately 15–20% of individuals over the age of 65 years old.[1] Over 100 000 peripheral vascular interventions are performed each year and, with the increasing incidence of peripheral vascular disease, peripheral interventions are also increasing. Approximately 10–15% of all percutaneous procedures are attempts at chronic total occlusion (CTO) recanalization.[2] Many approaches to total occlusions have been introduced, such as:

- PIER (percutaneous intentional extraluminal subintimal recanalization)
- the FlowCardia CROSSER system (currently pending approval), which works by introducing vibrational energy that provides mechanical impact and cavitational effects
- LuMend's Frontrunner device, which acts by blunt microdissections[2]
- the Tornus device, which acts by burrowing through the CTO while being used in conjunction with a guidewire
- the ILT Safe-Cross RF (radiofrequency) system, which will be the focus of this chapter.

ILT SAFE-CROSS RF SYSTEM

The ILT Safe-Cross RF system is a steerable fiberoptic guidewire system that is able to 'look forward', recognize arterial wall, and deliver RF energy to the CTO for the ultimate goal of recanalization.[3] It is based on the principle of optical low coherence reflectometry (OCR). The system is composed of an OCR unit, detachable catheter, and guidewire with the ability to deliver RF energy pulsations (Figures 19.1–19.3). The OCR unit consists of a sample and reference light source, 50/50 coupler, bandpass filter, and a demodulator. The fiberoptic wire illuminates in a forward direction; reflected light is then scanned and compared with the reflected known reference.[4] This scan occurs every half-second in the A scan mode of the system.[5] If the fiber's forward look is the arterial wall, a red light indicator will appear on the monitor and the operator will have no ability to deliver RF energy (Figure 19.4). If a CTO is encountered, a green light bar will illuminate, allowing the operator to perform RF ablation to the CTO. Fibrous tissue and disorganized plaque result in a reflective signal that decreases monotonically with increasing distance, unlike arterial wall, which consists of organized

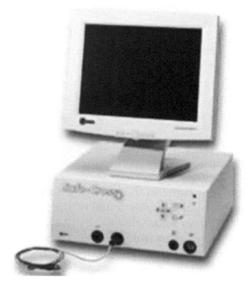

Figure 19.1   Safe-Cross console.

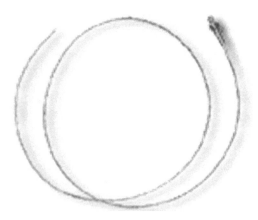

Figure 19.2 An 0.035 inch support catheter, 4.4 Fr.

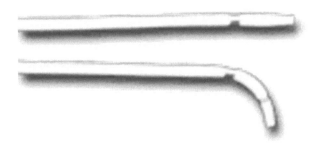

Figure 19.3   Two 0.014 inch straight and angled support catheters 3.0 Fr.

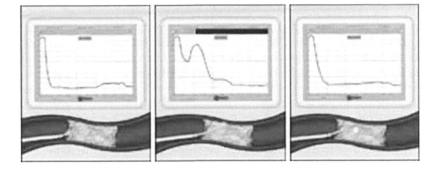

Figure 19.4   Console green indicates lumen, red indicates arterial wall.

tissue causing a secondary peak.[6] The wire is 275 cm in length and is capable of delivering energy between 200 and 500 kHz. Ablative energy is delivered in 20 millisecond bursts and the power discontinues after 20 seconds of continuous use, with the entire system being reset after a 3-second rest period. The Safe-Cross system offers straight or angled catheter tips. The Safe-Cross 0.014 inch support catheter system is a low-profile 3.0 Fr catheter system with straight or angled catheter tip for directionality (see Figure 19.3). The 0.035 inch support catheter system is a 4.4 Fr system with only a straight catheter tip (see Figure 19.2). Also available is a deflecting tip catheter, which comes in the 0.014 inch and 0.018 inch catheter sizes and is 3.5 and 4.0 Fr, respectively.

PHYSICS OF OPTICAL COHERENCE REFLECTOMETRY

Optical coherence reflectometry is a one-dimensional ranging method applied to studies in fiber-based waveguide devices.[7] Light is defined by its wavelength λ and frequency v, and spreads with different velocities within different media. These media-specific velocities allow for the differentiation between the different media. The intensity of the light wave is dependent on the interference of two light beams. When the phases of the two separate beams coincide, the beam of light is more intense; conversely, when the two beams are 180° out of phase, the light is canceled out. A more common scenario is that the beams may be slightly out of phase, causing the beam intensity to be diminished. This mixture of light waves is the functional basis of the optical inferometer used in the OCR system.

The OCR system (Figure 19.5) is based on the fiberoptic Michelson interferometer. A light source is fed through a 50/50 fiberoptic coupler and sent to a reference arm and to the sample. The light leaving the reference arm is focused at the reference mirror and the reflected light is collected by the reference fiber; similarly, the light leaving the sample arm is focused at the sample and the reflected light is collected by the sample fiber. Both backscattered lights are combined within the detector. In comparison to the reference mirror, the intensity of the optical beam produced by the two light sources is scanned in the detector, allowing for the differentiation of different depths. Differentiation of reflections can only occur when the difference of optical wavelengths between the light sources is within the coherence length of the light source. Coherence length of light is inversely proportional to its frequency. It is a measure of the coherence of the light beam. A high-coherent light source oscillates between the maximum and minimum amplitude, without much change as the reference light source is moved one-half optical wavelength. With a low-coherent optical beam system, source interference is only sensed when wavelengths of the sample and reference are closely matched to the coherence length of the light. This increase in resolution from a low-coherence system allows for better media differentiation. Currently, a resolution of 10 μm is commercially available.[8] Based on this mechanism, the OCR system is able to discriminate between lumen, CTO, and arterial wall.[9]

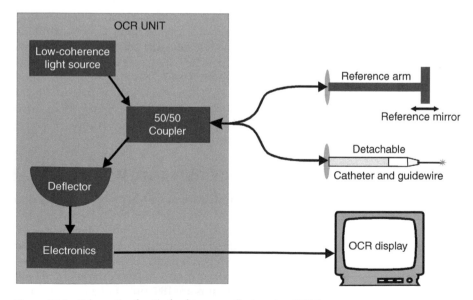

Figure 19.5 Schematic of optical coherence reflectometry (OCR) system.

GRIP TRIAL

The GRIP trial (usefulness of optical coherence reflectometry with guided radiofrequency energy to treat chronic total occlusions of peripheral arteries) was a multicenter prospective randomized study of the feasibility and safety of the ILT Safe-Cross device.[6] Fourteen sites throughout the USA enrolled 72 patients, with a total of 75 cases. All patients were known to have at least one chronic total occlusion in the native femoral, iliac, or popliteal artery of either lower extremity. Forty patients had contralateral groin access, with ipsilateral femoral, popliteal, or brachial access in 19 patients, and no available data for the remaining 13 patients. The average lesion length was 12.8 cm. A 6 Fr Bright Tip long sheath, 5 Fr Glide catheter, and Glidewire or Magic Torque wire were used. The operator was allowed a minimum of 10 minutes of fluoroscopic time, if at that time the operator was not able to cross the CTO in a conventional manner, ILT Safe-Cross system was used. Once confirmation of position was verified, ablative energy was administered at 200 Ω, at 3 W for low, 4 W for medium, and 5 W for high setting. Power was delivered in 20 ms bursts and RF ablation was disabled after 20 seconds of continuous use. Once the RF wire crossed the CTO, using the Glidecath and wire exchange techniques, traditional balloon angioplasty with or without stent placement was performed. Device success was defined as crossing of the CTO with the Safe-Cross catheter, whereas clinical success was defined as crossing of the CTO using any method. Among participants, clinical success and device success was achieved in 75% and 76% of all cases, respectively. Of the 57 cases that were crossed with the Safe-Cross device, 97% showed a decrease in the luminal area, with an average residual stenosis of 11%. There was no evidence of perforation or distal embolization, but a type C dissection was noted in one patient. Of the 57 lesions that were crossed, 90% were stented.

CASE REVIEW

We have used the ILT Safe-Cross RF system successfully in a number of patients with peripheral chronic total occlusions in whom previous attempts at revascularization had failed using conventional methods. We present the case of a 58-year-old female with a history of hypertension, dyslipidemia, and intractable claudication. Non-invasive studies demonstrated a bilateral ankle–brachial index (ABI) of 0.6. Chronic total occlusion of the left common iliac was treated with conventional percutaneous methods. The patient was also noted to have right external iliac total occlusion (Figure 19.6). A retrograde approach was initially attempted, with multiple wires such as the Glidewire, Cougar Wire, and the Magic Torque wire. This strategy was unsuccessful; therefore, a contralateral approach was utilized using a SOS OMNI catheter for contralateral access. This catheter and wire were then exchanged for the 0.035 inch RF wire and Safe-Cross catheter. The chronic occlusion was traversed and, using wire exchange techniques, a Glide catheter and Glidewire were positioned distal to the lesion. Angioplasty was then performed, with excellent results (Figure 19.8).

The second case is of a 76-year-old male with persistent claudication of his right lower leg for 5 years ABI.65. The pain had progressively worsened and the patient complained of rest leg pain. Arteriography demonstrated CTO of the

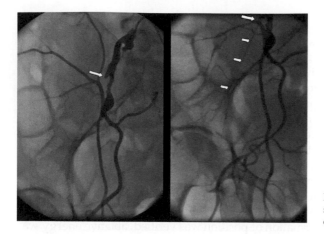

Figure 19.6 Arrow demonstrates the right external iliac chronic occlusion.

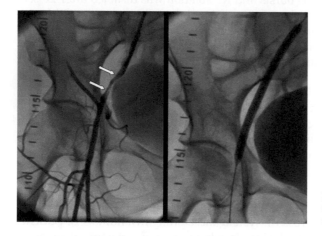

Figure 19.7 Arrow demonstrates initial stages of recanalization.

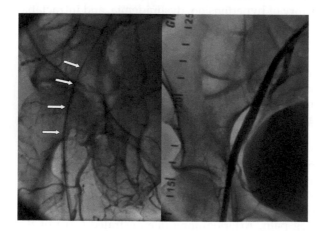

Figure 19.8 Arrow demonstrates angioplasty and the final result.

right popliteal artery (Figure 19.9). Conventional methods were initially attempted but after unsuccessfully crossing the CTO, the Safe-Cross catheter was used successfully. Angioplasty was performed without the need for stenting. The patient was claudication-free at follow-up. The lack of stenting was felt to be imperative in this patient, as the area of interest was at a flexion point. Stenting of flexion points has been fraught with complications such as stent fracture,[10]

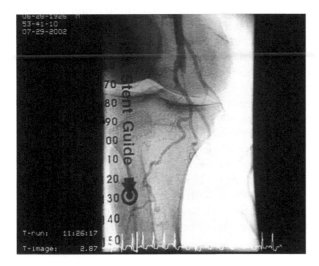

Figure 19.9 CTO of the popliteal artery.

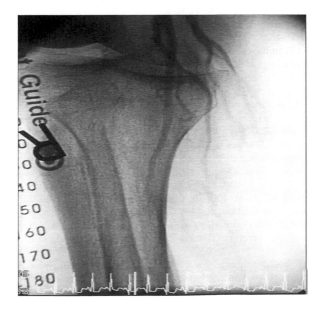

Figure 19.10 Recanalization of the popliteal artery.

pseudoaneurysm,[11] intramural hematoma,[12] and stent restenosis. The ILT Safe-Cross system assures the operator that he is truly in the lumen and no stent-requiring dissection has occurred.

CONCLUSION

Percutaneous options are often preferred by patients and their physicians because of the minimally invasive approach. This approach leads to expedited recovery, quicker time to ambulation, and the ability to preserve conduits, such as saphenous veins, for later possible use. As conventional percutaneous approaches to CTO recanalization have generally had a success rate of approximately 60%,[5] the ILT Safe-Cross RF system has proven to be a feasible alternative to these more conventional approaches, with success rates of 75–80% having been reported.[13] Also attractive is the safety profile, with reported rates of dissections and perforations being extremely low when using this system. Stenting CTOs at flexion points has the inherent risk of stent fracture and possible increase of in-stent restenosis. For this reason, at flexion points, in particular, the ILT Safe-Cross ensures advancement of the system within the lumen, eliminating stent-requiring dissections. Another appealing characteristic is the ease of use of the system, with green bars indicating 'go' and red indicating 'arterial wall', thus inhibiting the operator from delivering ablative energy to the wrong area and possibly causing coronary perforation. With its ease of use, safety profile, and high success rate, it is likely that the ILT Safe-Cross will continue to be a complimentary tool in the interventionalist's approach to CTOs.

REFERENCES

1. Hirsch AT, Haskal ZJ, Hertzer NR, et al. Practice Guidelines for the management of patients with peripheral arterial disease (lower extremity, renal, mesenteric, and abdominal aortic): a collaborative report. Circulation 2005; 113(11):e453–654.
2. Segev A, Strauss BH. Novel approaches for the treatment of chronic total coronary occlusions. J Interv Cardiol 2004; 17:411–16.
3. Ng W, Chen WH, Lee PY, Lau CP. Initial experience and safety in the treatment of chronic total coronary occlusions with a new optical coherent reflectometry-guided radiofrequency ablation guidewire. Am J Cardiol 2003; 92:732–4.
4. Huang D. Optical Coherence Tomography/Science, 1991; 254:1178–81.
5. Kirvaitis RJ, Heuser RR, Das TS, et al. Usefulness of optical coherent reflectometry with guided radiofrequency energy to treat chronic coronary total occlusions in peripheral arteries (the GRIP trial). Am J Cardiol 2004; 94:1081–4.
6. Baim DS, Braden G, Heuser RR, et al. Utility of the Safe-Cross-guided radiofrequency total occlusion crossing system in chronic coronary total occlusions (results from the Guided Radio Frequency Energy Ablation of Total Occlusions Registry). Am J Cardiol 2004; 94: 853–8.
7. Puma JA, Sketch MH Jr, Tcheng JE, et al. Percutaneous revascularization of chronic coronary occlusions: an overview. J Am Coll Cardiol 1995; 26: 1–11.
8. Shammas NW. Treatment of chronic total occlusions using optical coherent reflectometry and radiofrequency ablative energy: incremental success over conventional techniques. J Invasive Cardiol 2004; 16(2):58–9.
9. Wong P, Tse KK, Chan W. Recanalization of chronic total occlusion after conventional guidewire failure: guided by optical coherent reflectometry and facilitated by radiofrequency energy ablation. J Invasive Cardiol 2004; 16: 54–7.

10. Park SI, Won JH, Kim BM, Lee DY. The arterial folding point during flexion of the hip joint. Cardiovasc Intervent Radiol 2005; 28(2):173-7.
11. Solis J, Allaqaband S. A case of popliteal stent fracture with pseudoaneurysm formation. Catheter Cardiovasc Interv 2006; 67(2):319-22.
12. Maehara A, Mintz GS, Bui AB, et al. Incidence, morphology, angiographic findings, and outcomes of intramural hematomas after percutaneous coronary interventions: an intravascular ultrasound study. Circulation 2002; 105(17):2037-42.
13. Morales P, Kirvaitis R, Heuser R. Initial experience in the treatment of chronic superficial femoral artery occlusions with fiberoptic guidance technology. J Invasive Cardiol 2004; 16:485-8.

20

Tackling chronic total occlusions: training standards and recommendations

Ajay J Kirtane and George D Dangas

Cognitive skills required to approach revascularization of chronic total occlusions • Technical/procedural considerations and device-based training • CTO training within accredited interventional cardiology training programs • CTO-specific training and educational forums • Conclusions and proposed recommendations

Significant advances have been achieved in the ability to perform percutaneous coronary intervention (PCI) over the past several years through the use of advanced guidewire technologies, increasingly deliverable intracoronary balloon and stent platforms, and drug-eluting stents that greatly reduce the rates of restenosis. Despite these advances, the treatment of chronic total occlusions (CTO)s remains a labor-intensive process with procedural failure occurring in up to one-third of cases.[1,2] Thus, the successful treatment of CTOs is often referred to as the 'last frontier' of PCI, and operator experience is associated with greater rates of success in the therapy of these lesions.

Despite the fact that CTOs are frequently observed during routine diagnostic cardiac catheterization, PCI of CTOs is infrequently attempted, and CTOs are one of the most common lesion subsets referred for coronary artery bypass grafting (CABG); accordingly, this may be occurring with greater frequency for relatively inexperienced operators. Therefore, it is critical to establish educational curricula and practical training forums to help facilitate the process of advancing the operator skillset necessary to effect successful therapy of these lesions. In this chapter, we aim to illustrate some of the challenges faced in the successful treatment of these lesions and suggest CTO-specific training recommendations to aid the current and future generations of interventionalists in becoming facile in the treatment of these lesions.

COGNITIVE SKILLS REQUIRED TO APPROACH REVASCULARIZATION OF CHRONIC TOTAL OCCLUSIONS

CTOs are one of the most commonly observed lesion subsets during diagnostic cardiac catheterization, occurring in up to one-third of patients.[3] Nonetheless, only approximately 10–15% of patients with CTOs undergo percutaneous revascularization.[2] The decision-making of whether or not to proceed with PCI of a CTO is often complex, and is based upon the interplay of clinical patient-related considerations as well as more technical lesion-based factors. Technical issues related to the appearance of the CTO must be considered prior to attempting percutaneous recanalization of a CTO, as these can impact procedural success (Table 20.1). These include factors such as the age of the CTO, the length of the occlusion, the location of the occlusion (e.g. ostial vs in the body of the artery), the presence of a 'beak' without side branches, limited tortuosity and/or angulation of the artery, the presence of antegrade flow, and the presence of collaterals which can aid in the visualization of the distal vessel either antegrade or from the contralateral coronary artery.[1,4] Increased CTO technical ability through dedicated training can enhance the treatment options available.

Comprehensive appraisal

In our experience, the comprehensive appraisal of all these factors, even prior to performance of PCI for CTO, is not an inherently intuitive or algorithmic process, but rather is an acquired skill that is developed through operator experience over time. A familiarity with patient- and lesion-specific issues is critical in better determining which patients are candidates for revascularization, with a favorable chance of success and a low risk of complications. In addition, the comfort level of an operator with proceeding with CTO revascularization varies based upon individual experience, and another important factor is the commitment and support received from immediate colleagues or the collective practice group approach to percutaneous CTO revascularization. Even experienced operators occasionally find that CTO cases originally predicted to be rather straightforward may be difficult to recanalize, and similarly others that may have appeared to have a low likelihood of success are sometimes able to be crossed without significant difficulty. Collective practice experience can build a significant 'case library' of tips and tricks necessary for successful CTO recanalization.

A single common factor that appears to predict operator success of PCI for CTO is a 'incredible persistence' once the decision to intervene has been made, albeit without compromising the safety of the patient by knowing when to stop. At first, this may seem like a cognitive skill that can be taught and assimilated in the abstract (such as by reading this text, for example). However, in our experience, there is no substitute for the hands-on experience of interacting with an experienced operator and observing his/her thought process and approach to treating a CTO.

Table 20.1 Proposed lesion-specific guide for chronic total occlusions and anticipated success rates

	Recent total occlusion	CTO Level 1	CTO Level 2	CTO Level 3
Occlusion age	<3 months	3–6 months	6–12 months	>12 months
Angiographic features	Some thrombus or dye staining; TIMI 0–1 flow	Well-defined entry point, straight RCA or LAD, <10 mm length, no diffuse disease, distal vessel diameter easily visible, no major bridging collaterals	LCX occlusion, moderate tortuosity, 10–20 mm length, moderate calcification, bridging collaterals, intracoronary collaterals (neovasculature), patient age >80 years old or extensive peripheral disease, in-stent CTO >20 mm in length	Ostial occlusion without stump entry point, occlusion at takeoff of side branch, length >20 mm, occlusion in bend >60° or two bends of >45°, severe diffuse calcification, distal vessel course barely visible, tandem occlusion, occlusion that has been tried before unsuccessfully by experienced operator
Estimated procedural success	>90%	80–90%	70–80%	50–70%

CTO, chronic total occlusion; TIMI, Thrombolysis in Myocardial Infarction; RCA, right coronary artery; LAD, left anterior descending coronary artery; LCX, left circumflex coronary artery.
Adapted from Stone et al,[1] with permission.

TECHNICAL/PROCEDURAL CONSIDERATIONS AND DEVICE-BASED TRAINING

In addition to gaining CTO experience through appropriate case selection, it is important for the CTO interventionalist to be familiar with the latest technological advances and devices as well as intraprocedural techniques that may impact procedural success. A thorough knowledge of the latest developments in guide-wire construction is essential when deciding whether to employ stiffer, non-hydrophilic guidewires, which may be more useful in penetrating the proximal and distal ends of the fibrous cap of the CTO vs the appropriate scenarios for the use of a hydrophilic wire. In addition, familiarity with the use of specialized or novel devices can be useful in developing scenario-specific approaches to CTO revascularization (e.g. rotational atherectomy or other alternatives when balloon catheters cannot cross). These concepts are often taught at the fellowship level, or at more specialized/advanced technique-specific or device-specific forums.

Basic interventional techniques

First, there are basic required technical skills that may be more variably assimilated in training or in practice. A familiarity with over-the-wire techniques is critical in CTO revascularization, as this can directly impact the ability to transmit the force of the wire toward the CTO. Understanding the subtleties of guide catheter manipulation is another critical aspect of PCI of CTO, as larger and more anchored guiding catheters may not only be the deciding factor influencing the delivery of balloon catheters and stents once the CTO is crossed but may also lead to ostial dissections and compromised flow in other vessels (e.g. compromised flow to the circumflex from a deep-seated left coronary guide). In general, the initial CTO cases need to be performed with large French-size guiding catheters that provide significant passive support and with the operator being fully alert about possible guide-related complications and how to tackle them (large guiding catheters allow easier delivery of covered stents as well). With experience, smaller-size guiding catheters and active support with flexible guiding catheters or anchor balloon techniques can be used.

These types of basic interventional skills were more often required before the ascendancy of advances in rapid exchange technologies and the improvements in stent and balloon delivery systems and, in some ways, these techniques have become somewhat of a 'lost art'. Thus, it is critical to continue to emphasize their importance in training programs and in other forums such as live case demonstrations as a part of continuing medical education (CME).

Advanced techniques

Several more advanced procedural techniques have been described as being useful in facilitating successful PCI of CTOs, and operators wishing to fully embrace CTO revascularization should be familiar with their benefits and risks. For example, in our practice, we have found that relatively liberal use of dual injections (to allow visualization of the proximal and distal vessel in order to aid in guidewire manipulation) has been invaluable in impacting our success in CTO revascularization.

Other advanced techniques such as guide anchoring techniques, dual wire techniques (parallel wire, 'see-saw'), the retrograde approach via collaterals, intravascular ultrasound (IVUS)-based approach to CTOs, and the subintimal tracking and reentry (STAR) technique, are described in further detail elsewhere in this book and can be used selectively as required by the individual case.

We view a knowledge and familiarity with each of these techniques as essential in creating a comprehensive 'CTO toolbox' at the disposal of a CTO interventionalist. This toolbox, which can contain a full armamentarium of techniques and approaches to CTO recanalization, combined with clinical experience, is what separates the experienced CTO specialist from the casual CTO operator who may only have one or two guidewires and approaches at his/her disposal. Furthermore, it underlines the importance of nursing education in CTO and the contribution of the entire Cath Lab staff to timely performance of a successful CTO recanalization. Overall, there is a paucity of data that can clearly demonstrate the superiority of one methodology or approach over others, and it is the integration of a variety of approaches that in our opinion will have the highest likelihood of success.

Understanding CTO complications

In addition to gaining familiarity with techniques that can impact successful recanalization of a CTO, the responsible CTO interventionalist must possess knowledge of the management of complications that can occur during PCI for CTOs. PCI of CTOs is not without risk, and has been associated with an up to 3% incidence of adverse periprocedural complications.[1,5] Understanding and anticipating these complications is critical in the planning of a revascularization strategy. In addition to complications such as loss of side branches, compromise of collaterals, and dissections, CTO revascularization is also associated with high doses of radiation and contrast dye. Reducing radiation exposure through changing the beam angulation, coned-in images, lower magnification, and an awareness of total radiation dosing can help to minimize radiation-related complications. Adequate hydration and an awareness of total contrast dosage can potentially be useful in preventing contrast-related nephrotoxicity. Finally, meticulous attention to distal wire position, the exchange of aggressive wires for standard non-hydrophilic workhorse wires following successful catheter delivery to the distal vessel, and familiarity with needle pericardiocentesis and the use of covered stents and coils to treat perforations provides a higher level of safety during PCI of CTOs.

Exposure to novel techniques and devices

Despite recent advances in guidewire construction and the refinement of advanced CTO techniques, procedural success for CTO still lags far behind that of other PCI lesion subsets. As a result, the development of new devices and techniques for CTO is an area of active investigation. Exposure to these devices and technologies is often dependent upon the volume of individual PCI centers and/or exposure to animal-based device investigation. Interventionalists whose practice is based at these centers and trainees at these centers are afforded the unique opportunity to explore these technologies and form a base of experience with these technologies. Outside of these settings, however, even the 'early adopter' may be limited to device usage through enrollment in clinical trials and registries, and may additionally be somewhat dependent on industry contacts to foster exposure to new devices. The dissemination of these technologies beyond the major PCI centers and to the community interventionalist can be difficult, but is of critical importance.

CTO TRAINING WITHIN ACCREDITED INTERVENTIONAL CARDIOLOGY TRAINING PROGRAMS

Due to the combination of complexity and relative rarity, CTO techniques cannot be easily taught in full within the 1-year fellowship in interventional cardiology. In addition, the minority of fellowship graduates will probably be faced with several CTO lesions shortly after completion of the fellowship. Therefore, the main goal of fellowship training would be to impart the cognitive decision-making process regarding initiating a CTO attempt, the favorable and unfavorable characteristics, the technical and procedural risks, and ways to avoid or treat them. Such instruction can be given mainly through didactic sessions, case reviews, or quality assurance conferences.

Hands-on training can be initiated gradually during the second part of the accredited fellowship with the main goal of setting the stage for further development of skills during the next career steps (should it be necessary). Mastering CTO techniques should be viewed at this time as a more demanding subspecialty that, at this point, would be primarily driven by the needs of the individual clinical practice (i.e. similar to peripheral, carotid, aortic, valvular, structural, or congenital heart disease).

CTO-SPECIFIC TRAINING AND EDUCATIONAL FORUMS

Although intensive case review and exposure to the complexity of clinical, procedural, and device-based considerations mentioned above are generally a requisite part of high-volume fellowship training programs, they may not exist outside of this setting for other trainees, or for interventionalists currently in practice who attempt a limited number of CTO interventions. Specific CTO-based training sessions and CME forums may have the ability to serve as surrogates for intensive CTO-based fellowship training for these operators.

Fellowship training

Fellowship training in interventional cardiology is typically constructed as an apprenticeship with didactic components via lectures and conferences. With the renewed interest and advances in CTO revascularization options, successful fellowship training programs must emphasize not only didactics dedicated to CTO revascularization but also must make an effort to promote the teaching of practical CTO-based PCI skills to trainees. A simple reemphasis on many basic techniques such as wire selection, guide management, and the use of over-the-wire systems can be invaluable to trainees who may otherwise have received limited teaching or had insufficient exposure to these issues. Advanced techniques in CTO revascularization can often be learned through the apprenticeship model (by observing experienced operators within the training institution) and can be supplemented by observing live case demonstrations at conferences or other CME-based forums.

CTO-specific training after fellowship

For the interventionalist currently in practice who may not be exposed to specific CTO-based teaching in training, several CTO-based sessions are already available both as separate meetings and/or as a subcomponent of major interventional meetings. The didactics and live case demonstrations at these meetings are in general very favorably viewed and can be invaluable additions to clinical practice experience of these interventionalists. These meetings can also serve to provide exposure to newer devices and the cutting edge in novel techniques.

On a smaller scale, as the field of CTO revascularization continues to advance, the opportunity for individual 'CTO training days' should present intensive opportunities for more case-based and face-to-face learning. One could envision a 1–2 day course where a small group of interventionalists observe and assist a senior and experienced CTO operator in a number of CTO cases in succession. These types of sessions could foster the further development of the cognitive skills of case selection while allowing further hands-on experience with novel devices and techniques.

Simulation training

Simulation programs have at this point not been specifically designed to aid in CTO-based training, but may offer many advantages in the future since they have the fundamental components to assist in practical education in this area. These programs can be used to aid in the introduction of operators to novel wires, devices, and advanced techniques in a 'risk-free' environment. Additionally, simulation programs offer the unique ability to troubleshoot and treat complications that can occur during CTO revascularization. Whereas CTO revascularization is associated with a higher rate of complications than revascularization of less-complex lesions, the overall complication rate is still relatively low. Thus, simulators can allow operators to experience and treat different (and even rare) complications without having to attempt PCI of a CTO in hundreds of live patients and without the consequences of a complication in a live patient. Although clinical scenarios presented at a simulation course may to some extent lack the reality of actual patient contact, they can serve as a forum for discussion and thought and, particularly for trainees or even for more experienced interventionalists not commonly exposed to the breadth of CTO revascularization options, they can serve as an invaluable proxy for clinical experience in the management of these patients.

CONCLUSIONS AND PROPOSED RECOMMENDATIONS

Revascularization of CTOs is an advanced PCI technique that requires the operator to integrate a variety of cognitive and technical skills in order to proceed

Table 20.2   Proposed CTO training standards

Didactic courses
1. [a]CTO background: pathophysiology of atherosclerosis/histopathology of CTOs, clinical presentation, natural history, and rationale for treatment
2. [a]CTO guidewire design, guide management, and over-the-wire techniques
3. Advanced CTO techniques
4. [a]CTO complications and management (technical as well as radiation exposure and contrast nephrotoxicity)
5. Novel CTO devices

[a]Case-based training standards: 10 CTO cases with case review performed per year (primary operator or assistant to an experienced primary operator)

CME: attendance at CTO-based training sessions or simulation every 1–2 years

[a]Can generally be achieved during part of ACGME-accredited interventional cardiology fellowship training program.
CTO, chronic total occlusion; CME, continuing medical education; ACGME, Accreditation Council for Graduate Medical Education.

successfully and safely, while at the same time imparting prognostic benefit to the patient. Therefore, it is essential for the basic and advanced components of CTO revascularization to be taught in both a didactic and hands-on manner to operators wishing to further pursue CTO revascularization. In our opinions, training standards for CTO revascularization can help to ensure the highest level of operator expertise for this advanced PCI technique. Examples of these proposed standards are illustrated in Table 20.2.

In summary, the renewed emphasis upon PCI-based CTO revascularization must be met with a renewed emphasis on CTO-based training and teaching. Without an interest in the development and dissemination of specific CTO-based skills and training, CTO revascularization will remain relegated to an obscure and mysterious art, understood by some and awed by many.

REFERENCES

1. Stone GW, Colombo A, Teirstein PS, et al. Percutaneous recanalization of chronically occluded coronary arteries: procedural techniques, devices, and results. Catheter Cardiovasc Interv 2005; 66:217–36.
2. Stone GW, Kandzari DE, Mehran R, et al. Percutaneous recanalization of chronically occluded coronary arteries: a consensus document: part I. Circulation 2005; 112:2364–72.
3. Kahn JK. Angiographic suitability for catheter revascularization of total coronary occlusions in patients from a community hospital setting. Am Heart J 1993; 126:561–4.
4. Stone GW, Reifart NJ, Moussa I, et al. Percutaneous recanalization of chronically occluded coronary arteries: a consensus document: part II. Circulation 2005; 112:2530–7.
5. Suero JA, Marso SP, Jones PG, et al. Procedural outcomes and long-term survival among patients undergoing percutaneous coronary intervention of a chronic total occlusion in native coronary arteries: a 20-year experience. J Am Coll Cardiol 2001; 38:409–14.

Index

Note: Page references in *italics* refer to Figures and Tables

T - #0127 - 111024 - C250 - 234/156/12 - PB - 9780367452957 - Gloss Lamination